Woman's Day's 1000 Questions About Women's Health

Woman's Day's 1000 Questions About Women's Health

Nancy G. Brinker

and

H. Jane Chihal, M.D., Ph.D.

THE SUMMIT PUBLISHING GROUP
Arlington, Texas

THE SUMMIT PUBLISHING GROUP
One Arlington Centre, 1112 East Copeland Road, Fifth Floor
Arlington, Texas 76011
summit@dfw.net
www.summitbooks.com

This book is not intended to be a substitute for professional medical advice. The reader should regularly consult a physician regarding any matter concerning her health, especially in reagrd to any symptoms that might require diagnosis or medical attention. Medical science is an ever-changing field. Every effort has been made to ensure that the medical information contained in this book was the most accurate and current at the time of publication. Any mention in this book of actual products sold does not constitute an endorsement by the publisher or the author, except where noted. This book does not establish a physician-patient relationship. The authors, publisher, and Women's Day Magazine, disclaim any liability either direct or indirect which results from adherence to any advice contained within or actions taken because of, this text.

Copyright © 1997 by The Summit Publishing Group

All rights reserved. No part of this book may be reproduced or transmitted in any form or by any means, electronic or mechanical, including photocopying, recording, or by any information storage and retrieval system, without the written permission of the publisher, except where permitted by law.

Printed in the United States of America.

01 00 99 98 97 010 5 4 3 2 1

Library of Congress Cataloging-in-Publication Data

Brinker, Nancy.
Woman's day's 1,000 questions about women's health / Nancy Brinker and H. Jane Chihal.
p. cm.
Includes index.
ISBN 1-56530-272-9 (pbk.)
1. Women--Health and hygiene--Miscellanea. I. Chihal, H. Jane.
II. Title. III. Title: Woman's day's one thousand questions about women's health.
RA778.B83 1997
613'.04244--dc21
97-33783
CIP

Cover design by Gary Templin
Book design by Chris Robinson
Writing support by Eileen Marin
Index by Michael Rossa

To the women who are not afraid to ask and the doctors who are not afraid to answer

Table of Contents

Foreword

Attitudes about healthcare have undergone enormous changes in recent years. For generations, the prevailing wisdom was essentially "fix it if it breaks." In the last few decades, however, we've come to realize that healthcare actually begins long *before* something goes wrong. Taking care of mind and body is ongoing, and it's up to each of us to take an active role in the endeavor.

That's exactly what's behind this book, and we at *Woman's Day* are proud to be part of it. Our commitment to covering women's health issues is longstanding, as this edition attests. It was conceived as a straightforward, easy-to-use guide to the unique health issues women face today, and we are confident that it will prove an invaluable resource. We are also deeply indebted to its authors, Dr. Jane Chihal, a practicing physician, and Nancy Brinker, one of the nation's leading patient advocates. They bring years of experience to these pages and their expertise is unparalleled.

Read in good health.

Jane Chesnutt
Editor-in-Chief
Woman's Day

Preface

Nancy Brinker

Questions are important, so go ahead and ask them! They'll make you a more educated consumer of health-care information when you really need it–when you or someone you care about is a patient. I know many of you are embarrassed to ask them, and even more of us (notice the us) are too confused to know what to ask. Indeed, forming the question is sometimes the hardest part.

Immediately following that, though, is sitting still long enough to listen to the answer. How many times have you sat on one of those cold doctor's office tables in a silly gown that makes you feel more like a specimen than a human and tried to listen to the doctor rattle off a series of comments? You're uncomfortable and you hardly heard a word the doctor said. That's where this book comes in.

Over the years I've asked lots of questions. Not only for myself, but also for my family, friends, and complete strangers who have asked me to help them figure out what it is they need to know. The question-and-answer format of this book allows me to speak for you, the women who have asked me questions for over twenty years. I asked the doctor your questions, and she responded in straightforward, easy-to-understand language. Remember, this book is intended to be educational but is not a substitute for a medical exam or diagnosis.

I am proud that I have had the opportunity to do the work that I have done over the years. I hope that through this book I will once again reach out to people to help them shape their concerns and feel comfortable asking questions of their doctors, nurses, and other caregivers so that each of them can be a part of a solution.

In 1996, I was lucky enough to meet and work with Dr. Jane Chihal at a conference. I was taken with her low-key yet knowledgeable style of communication and the fact that she cared enough to write on a variety of health issues. I believe that our united efforts result in two plus two equaling five. I thank Jane for doing an outstanding job in answering these questions, and in being there as a true partner in this effort.

To my good friend and business partner Jeff Zucker, thanks for making all this possible!

I also want to give tremendous thanks to the editor of this book, Eileen Marin, who has done an absolutely outstanding job in helping us put shape to this message. Quite simply, without Eileen this book would not exist.

Over the years, there have been so many people who have helped me to help others. To my parents, Marvin and Ellie Goodman; my son, Eric; my cousins, Cindy, Mark, and Nancy; my step-daughters, Brenda and Cindy; and to Doris, Ela, Andy, Alexandra, Barbie, and Margaret. I never get to say enough how much I appreciate and respect you as people, family, and friends.

And then there is Norman. You are the answer to my prayers.

Nancy

Jane Chihal, M.D., Ph.D., F.A.C.O.G.

For almost twenty years I have dedicated my professional life to providing comprehensive medical care for women. My concept of working as a partner with each patient to provide individualized, proactive, preventive medical care has gradually evolved as I have grown and matured as a physician and as a woman. The key to making this partnership work is an informed patient and a well-trained physician—two people who are willing to communicate effectively. The partnership concept implies equal responsibility; the physician must evaluate each patient and offer options, and the woman must make decisions and manage her own health care.

Women must learn to critically evaluate medical news. Anecdotal stories about the success of treatments are no substitute for data based on scientific information. Everyone looks for the answers they want to hear. Physicians and patients alike must keep an open mind in their search for the truth.

This book has been an opportunity for me to provide factual, easy-to-read information on women's health care, and empower women to select a health-care provider to meet their needs and form their own effective health-care partnership.

I am grateful to Nancy Brinker, who believes in the physician-patient partnership, for offering me this opportunity to work with her. Nancy truly is our health and wellness champion. We come together through this book, as a physician and health-care advocate, to encourage women everywhere to seek health-care relationships that will nourish their lives. Don't ever settle for less.

H Jane Chihal, M.D.

Part I

Understanding Today's Health-Care System

1

A Conversation with Nancy and Jane

1

N: It's been important for me to help educate women to be proactive in their health care, to learn how to find, and then partner with, a physician. Choosing a doctor who fits a woman's needs, finances, and the parameters of health insurance is difficult today. Women need to learn to trust their judgment when they feel a health-care provider is making light of a concern or listening half heartedly. Everyone deserves to be heard. How do you feel when someone comes in and starts questioning your experience and credentials?

J: I think asking the right questions before you choose a doctor is important. The informed patient should ask about the doctor's education, experience, and whether they are board certified. The woman should continue her search if the physician is uncomfortable with the questions or feels threatened. The doctor has to be open and willing to partner with a patient to form a team. The patient can be assertive and ask for things she wants and needs as long as it is done in a considerate rather than confrontational manner. Like any successful relationship, there has to be give and take on both sides.

2

N: The Patients Bill of Rights is posted in hospitals, and I've seen it in a number of doctors' offices. What protection does it give us?

J: There are many different versions of the Patients Bill of Rights. They all include quality care for all patients regardless of race, creed, color, sex, age, disability, or financial status. Patients should have fully informed consent, which means they should be told what procedures will be performed and the risks of treatments they will receive. They have the right to request a transfer to another facility, refuse treatment, and be informed if they will be included in an experimental treatment. Patients also have the right to privacy, dignity, confidentiality, and access to their medical records.

3

N: In times of crisis, or when a variety of things are going on at one time, it's hard to remember everything. I often suggest women take a tape recorder with them to the doctor for that very reason. Would you have a problem if a patient walked in for her appointment with a tape recorder?

J: I encourage patients to take notes during their visits. I also suggest after surgery that family members tape record our conversations. The patient can then hear what I said when he or she comes out of anesthesia. Some physicians are going to feel threatened by a tape recorder because they are unsure how the information will be used. Assurance that it is for personal use only may alleviate some of the concerns. If the tape recording is especially important, check with the physician's office staff before the appointment to see if it is permitted.

4

N: Whatever happened to the doctors we grew up with? I often hear women say their doctors are victims of a "time clock mentality." What do you think is happening to the old bedside manner, the personal care our parents were used to?

J: Physicians feel a lot of stress from managed care companies that seem to be dictating how to treat patients. Most are expected to see more people, in less time, with more restrictions, for less money. Not only do we have to keep up with the latest drugs and procedures, but we are also constantly doing battle with administrators, codes, and rules imposed by insurance companies. A lot of the enjoyment of direct patient care has been eroded by the fight to survive in a new kind of medicine.

5

N: What type of training does a person receive before he or she can start practicing medicine?

J: Generally, medical school is a four full years past a college degree. Most states then require at least one year of postgraduate training as an intern before they will give someone a medical license. Many physicians choose to go on to some type of specialty training. A residency can vary between two and five additional years after an internship.

6

N: What does it mean for a physician to be board certified?

J: Board Certification by the American Board of Approved Specialties shows that a physician has completed an approved medical school and an approved residency program in a specific specialty and has passed both written and oral examinations. Having a Board Certification doesn't guarantee they are the best in their field, but it does indicate they have passed a competency test of their peers. Any other board licensing does not stand the rigors of Board Certification.

7

N: What's the difference between a D.O. and an M.D.?

J: A D.O. is a Doctor of Osteopathy and an M.D. is a Medical Doctor. Both take boards and are licensed by the same or similar agencies. Both treat the same illnesses, prescribe medications, and perform surgery. Many of the treatments they use are similar. Years ago, there was a definitive difference in their philosophies toward illness. The Doctor of Osteopathy incorporates alternative treatments into his or her practice more frequently than the Medical Doctor. Medical Doctor treatments are based more on traditional, Western scientific data.

8

N: People who live in small cities, or rural areas, often have one medical provider that treats all of their needs. Living in a big city we see nurse clinicians, nurse practitioners, physician's assistants, and even midwives. What's the difference between all of them?

J: There are many well-trained health professionals that can extend the reach of the physician. A nurse clinician or practitioner is a registered nurse with eighteen to twenty-four months of additional training. He or she may work as a team member with a physician to provide preventive care and treatment of uncomplicated medical illnesses. A physician's assistant has completed a two-year program and works directly under the supervision of a physician to evaluate and treat patients. Midwives are nurses with special training in the care of pregnant women and uncomplicated births.

9

N: The National Institutes of Health has a department of alternative medicine that is studying new treatments. Many other facilities and organizations are evaluating the effectiveness of plants and herbs in healing. There seems to be a quest for alternatives to toxic medications. Is there a place for these alternatives in Western medicine?

J: We still know very little about herbal medicine and other alternative therapies. Undoubtedly, some of these are beneficial. Most are not dangerous, but some can be toxic to the body. Traditional medicine must be open to new ideas and scientifically study these alternative approaches to healing. Many currently used medications were originally formulated from herbal medicines, such as opium and digitalis.

10

N: Why does it take so long for doctors to be able to prescribe new medications we read about in magazines?

J: The information age is presenting medical information to the public faster than the completion of a variety of accurate medical studies. History is full of published studies, from reputable laboratories, that were found to be incorrect when repeated. The media often reports information before the actual journal findings reach a physician's desk. Even after studies are conducted and deemed reliable, the government has stringent rules before a medication can be prescribed to a patient.

11

N: The way the price of medications has escalated through the years is shocking. Why are they so expensive?

J: It can cost over two hundred million dollars to develop a single new drug and get it approved through the Food and Drug Administration. A patent lasts for nineteen years and starts during the development stage of a drug. If it takes ten years to develop the drug, the exclusive patent is only good for nine additional years. The company has to make enough money to cover the cost of development, fund new research, and make a profit. All of this filters down to customers when they pay the pharmacy.

12

N: How do I know if an organization I donate money to is using it effectively to help improve women's health care?

J: It's important to ask the management staff at a particular organization where your dollar is actually being spent. Find out how much is committed to research, grants, and administrative expenses.

13

N: There are so many medications that are now over-the-counter that required a prescription years ago. How do we decide when to treat ourselves and when to go to a doctor?

J: It is a good idea to talk with the pharmacist about over-the-counter remedies if you're having a minor problem. The pharmacist is a highly trained professional and a good source of information about over-the-counter medications. If symptoms are not relieved in a reasonable time, say one to two weeks, you should see a physician for an evaluation.

14

N: What should a patient do if she thinks her physician is abusing alcohol or drugs?

J: Although most abusers are in denial about their use, I suggest you begin by saying something to the physician. Be sure of your concerns and facts before making any official accusations. If your physician has been awake for many hours for an emergency, she or he may show signs of sleep deprivation, which can mimic substance abuse behavior. A patient can contact the chief of staff or hospital administrator where the doctor has privileges. There is a Physician Activities Committee that will investigate. Or you can write or call the State Board of Medical Examiners or the County Medical Society and let them know about your concerns.

15

N: How does a nonmedical person know what to trust and what to ignore when reading an article or report that appears in a journal, magazine, or newsletter?

J: There are several factors to look for in an authentic article. It's important to see who sponsors the journal; is it the American Medical Association (AMA) or a Dictionary of Herbs that no one ever heard of? Check the author and her credentials. If she or he is quoting a study, see how many people participated and if there was a control group. It's important that the study be blinded, that is, neither the patient nor physician knew who took the real drug or the placebo. Anecdotal or individual stories make interesting reading but have no scientific value. It's always good to ask your physician for an opinion on what appears in the press.

16

N: How reliable is the medical information we access on the Internet?

J: Just like everything else, some information comes from highly reliable sources while other information, which may look like scientifically based data, is really advertising. Finding it on the Internet, or in any printed material for that matter, doesn't make it true. Again, evaluate the source of the information and discuss it with your physician.

17

N: Can you explain the difference between an HMO and a PPO?

J: An HMO is a health maintenance organization. There is usually a primary-care physician who serves as a sort of gatekeeper. She or he must follow certain guidelines to refer the patient for tests or evaluation by a specialist. There are rarely out-of-network benefits. The PPO is a preferred provider organization, which is comprised of physicians who have an agreement to provide services for their insured. Some PPOs do provide out-of-network benefits. In these instances, a patient can go to a doctor outside of the preferred provider network, but the PPO will pay a smaller percentage of the doctor's fee. For example, the PPO may 90 percent of an office visit with a doctor in the network and only 70 percent of an office visit with a doctor outside of the network.

18

N: Can a patient file a protest if she experiences a problem with a PPO or HMO?

J: If there is a disagreement with the insurance carrier, the problem should be discussed with the primary-care physician. If this does not resolve the issue, an appeal can be made to the medical director of the insurance company or to the company's committee that considers grievances. Contact the State Board of Insurance if there continues to be no resolution to the problem.

19

N: It took me a long time to understand the managed care system. Is there an easy way to describe capitation to someone not familiar with the term?

J: Capitation is a new form of insurance whereby the physician agrees to accept a fixed payment from the insurance company for treating patients. The doctor is paid the same amount whether he or she actually treats the patient or has no contact for that particular year. The goal is to limit the liability of the insurance company. Using this type of arrangement, there is no financial motivation for the physician to offer the patient additional evaluation or treatment. In fact, the physician may be penalized for ordering "too many" tests or medications. There is concern about capitation as a way of limiting costs while compromising the best interests of the patients. If you are shopping for an insurance company, you should ask them whether or not they employ capitation.

20

N: How does an insurance company's preferred drug list alter what medications a doctor might prescribe?

J: Insurance companies want physicians to consider the cost in addition to the effectiveness of medications they prescribe. For example, ampicillin is an inexpensive, safe antibiotic for the treatment of ear infections. However, it doesn't cure about 25 percent of the bacteria that cause ear infections. Instead of prescribing a more expensive antibiotic that cures more ear infections, the insurance company may require the physician to prescribe ampicillin first and then re-treat the failures with the more expensive drug.

21

N: Who runs a hospital and determines the quality of care for the patients?

J: The hospital can be administered by a commercial organization or a nonprofit board of directors. The employees of the hospital, from the janitors to the nurses, are hired and supervised by the company or board that runs the hospital. The physician staff admits patients to the hospital and determines the medical policies the hospital should follow.

22

N: How do hospitals decide which doctors will be allowed to perform surgery or other procedures at their facilities?

J: The medical staff of the hospital evaluates the application of each health-care professional who wants to practice in its institution. It is its responsibility to determine that each professional has the training, skills, and judgment to perform his or her duties. This is an ongoing process with regular evaluations for each physician.

23

N: How does a hospital staff discipline a physician?

J: Every hospital has a formal group, usually appointed by the president of the medical staff, that investigates an allegation and makes a report to the executive committee. Physicians who have been shown to practice inappropriate medicine or poor judgment can have their privileges restricted or even revoked.

24

N: How does a woman choose the best physician for herself and her family?

J: It is best to select a physician based on reputation in the community, training, and patient communication skills. If forced to work within the confines of an insurance plan, make a list of what the family is looking for from a physician. Then select names from the insurance program list who are in a close geographic location. Call the physicians' offices and request a brief interview on the phone or in person or a short bio including educational background. Ask for referrals from friends and family members. In addition, contact the local hospital as another referral source.

25

N: Why are doctors so worried about being sued?

J: Like anyone else, a doctor can be wrongly sued. Even a groundless suit can cost thousands of dollars and weeks away from the office in legal proceedings. Patients want their doctors to be perfect, but they are only human beings. Practicing defensive medicine isn't good for anyone. Most physicians, however, are still trying to take the best care of their patients without the fear of lawsuits on their mind.

26

N: What should someone do if they become ill away from home?

J: If they are in the United States, they should contact the county medical society, ask their hotel for a recommendation, or call the local hospital. The U.S. embassy, hotel, or a credit card company should be contacted for a referral outside of the country.

Part II
The Phases of Life

2

Puberty

27

Q What is puberty?

A Puberty is the gradual process that physically turns a girl into a woman capable of reproducing. Emotional maturity doesn't necessarily develop at the same rate. The first physical sign of puberty is usually breast budding. The nipple of the breast starts to extend beyond the chest wall. Then gradually the tissue under the nipple increases to push the nipple forward in a cone shape. The rounded shape of the mature breast doesn't occur until much later. A few coarse pubic hairs begin to appear shortly after breast development. It is at the end of puberty that her menstrual cycle will begin.

28

Q What do you tell a young girl who feels like she's the only one in the whole world, or at least her school, who doesn't wear a bra?

A Every girl goes through puberty in her own time. If your daughter isn't showing signs of breast development by the age of fourteen, you should take her to the doctor for an evaluation. Girls who are short and thin, especially if they are athletic, go through puberty late. Girls who are taller and heavier are often early bloomers. Share some of your history and reassure your daughter that there is a wide variation of normal growth.

29

Q When should a girl expect to start her first menstrual cycle?

A Most girls will start their menstrual cycles between two and two and a half years after breast budding begins. By noting the start of breast development, you will be able to determine the approximate time of her first period (menses). This information will allow you time to prepare your daughter for this normal life event.

30

Q Is it normal for a thirteen-year-old girl to have irregular menstrual cycles?

A The rhythm of menstrual cycles is controlled by egg release (ovulation), which occurs about fourteen days prior to the onset of a period. Egg release often fails in the first year or two. It's as if the reproductive system has to practice to regulate all of the complicated hormone interactions that must occur for estrogen production, egg release, and preparation of the uterine lining for a possible pregnancy. It is common to have a period every two to six weeks or skip a cycle in that first year or two. If the irregularity does not correct itself, if there's heavy bleeding, or if there's significant pain unrelieved by over-the-counter medications, consult your health-care professional.

31

Q Is it okay for a teenager to use tampons?

A Teenagers can use tampons if they wish. The vaginal opening is large enough for most girls to be able to insert a tampon without discomfort. Wearing tampons has nothing to do with virginity. Using a small or junior tampon with a light coating of petroleum jelly often helps her learn the insertion technique. She should read the package directions carefully and wash her hands before inserting the tampon. If she has trouble, she should see a gynecologist or nurse practitioner for help.

32

Q Is toxic shock syndrome from tampons a threat to teenage girls?

A Toxic shock is a rare disorder caused by a toxin produced by a staph bacteria. Concerns about toxic shock should not stop a woman from using tampons. However, certain precautions should be taken. It's important to wash hands with soap and water prior to tampon insertion and use the smallest tampon that is adequate for the menstrual flow (don't use a super tampon on a light day). Make sure tampons are changed at least three times a day. If a rash and high fever develop while using tampons, remove the tampon and call a physician.

33

Q Is it cause for concern if a teenage girl notices one of her breasts is larger than the other?

A On careful inspection, most women will notice one breast is larger than the other. However, this difference in size is more significant during breast development. If a marked difference in breast size (asymmetry) continues for several years after menses, a plastic surgeon should be consulted. Reassurance is usually the best therapy, but if a case is particularly severe, a custom foundation shop can suggest a bra that will optimize her appearance in clothes.

34

Q What's the best way for a teenage girl to treat menstrual cramps?

A Mild to moderate menstrual cramps are common. They are caused by the release from the uterine lining of prostaglandins, which stimulate muscle contractions or cramps. Often over-the-counter pain medications, such as ibuprofen (found in Advil) or naproxen sodium (found in Aleve), are effective in relieving the discomfort of cramps. These medications work better if the woman starts them prior to the actual onset of her period. It is important to take the medication with a full glass of fluid and at least a little food to help protect the stomach from irritation. Continue to take as directed until the end of menses. Cramps will return if the medications are stopped too early. Some discomfort can be expected during menses, but no one should be told it is "normal" to have pain severe enough to cause vomiting or to require bedrest. Birth control pills are sometimes prescribed to improve menstrual cramps. See your health-care professional for severe cramps not relieved by the over-the-counter medications.

35

Q When should you talk to a young girl about sex?

A These questions often start when your child is three or four years old. The answers get more complicated as the years go by. Kids are curious and will ask questions as long as they aren't embarrassed or repressed. Give short, direct answers to the questions they ask. Don't provide more information than is asked for, because they will ask more detailed questions as they are able to understand the information. The American College of Obstetrics and Gynecology has an excellent pamphlet called *Growing Up*. Your physician can order it for you.

36

Q What do you recommend telling teenagers about birth control?

A Information on birth control will not encourage a teenager to be promiscuous. Numerous studies have shown that lack of birth control information increases teenage pregnancy. Birth control information, especially the use of condoms, which may decrease the risks of sexually transmitted diseases (STDs), should be provided by eleven years of age. There is nothing wrong with providing factual information while encouraging abstinence. You don't get pregnant or get an STD if you don't have sex. Keeping a line of communication open with your teenager and encouraging decisions based on family moral values will help her resist peer pressure to be sexually active in high school.

37

Q When should a girl go to a gynecologist?

A It's a good idea for a teenage girl to visit with a gynecologist before any problems arise. A talk with your health provider ahead of time will smooth the way for a discussion and exam that excludes a pelvic later on. Reassure your daughter the visit will not include a pelvic exam but she will learn how to perform a breast self-exam and be able to ask the doctor questions. At a later visit, an initial well-woman pelvic examination can be done. Other reasons she may visit would be if she were experiencing severe menstrual cramps that are unrelieved by over-the-counter medications, persistent irregular bleeding, pelvic pain, failure to start breast development by age fourteen or menses by sixteen, milky discharge or other fluid from the breast (galactorrhea), abnormal vaginal discharge, or to get birth control and STD counseling.

38

Q Is it dangerous for a teenager to take birth control pills?

A Once a young woman has had her first menses, oral contraceptives are very safe and effective. Birth control pills do not increase the risk of future infertility. Unless a woman is in a long-term, monogamous relationship, she should use condoms to prevent sexually transmitted diseases in addition to taking the pill. There are many noncontraceptive benefits of the pill including control of irregular cycles, decrease in menstrual cramps (dysmenorrhea), decrease in abnormal hair growth (hirsutism), increase in bone strength, and improvement in acne problems. Furthermore, if a woman takes the pill for more than eight years during her lifetime, she decreases her risk of ovarian cancer by 80 percent. Women with irregular cycles decrease their risk of endometrial (uterine) cancer if they take the pill.

39

Q Is there something wrong with a second grader showing signs of sexual development?

A Most of the time precocious or early puberty poses no harm to the development of the child. It may, however, cause some social problems because she stands out from the other girls. Early activation of puberty can be treated with medication to reverse the symptoms. Those who start puberty early are initially tall but end up short as adults. Reversal of precocious puberty allows the bones to grow more, resulting in greater height. There are, however, some serious problems, such as tumors, that can cause early sexual development. If your child starts sexual development prior to the age of seven and a half, a pediatrician or an endocrinologist should be consulted.

40

Q Is there something wrong with a sixteen-year-old girl who seems happy and active but hasn't started her menstrual cycle?

A The onset of menses can be delayed by too little body fat. A certain amount of fat is necessary for normal menses and fertility. Long-distance runners, ballerinas, and other female athletes may start their periods late. Women suffering from eating disorders such as anorexia nervosa or bulimia commonly start their periods late or have a normal puberty but have a reversal of sexual maturity and stop having cycles. An evaluation by a physician will rule out serious problems.

41

Q Should teenage girls take calcium supplements?

A Most teenagers don't get enough calcium in their diet from food. A girl should get at least 1,000 mg daily. A supplement is easier than trying to change her diet. Encourage her to take 400 mg of calcium citrate in the morning. Calcium citrate can be absorbed on an empty stomach. Chewing a Tums tablet two or three times daily with a meal works as does calcium-fortified orange juice. The skeleton doesn't reach maximum strength until the age of thirty-five. The stronger the bones are by then, the less risk of osteoporosis later on.

42

Q Why are young girls often so much taller than boys their age?

A There is a marked growth spurt during puberty for both girls and boys. However, girls enter puberty at a younger age than boys. Therefore, most girls are taller than the boys at the end of elementary school. Most girls reach their maximum height by age fifteen while the boys don't start to accelerate until that time. Remember that everyone matures on their own timetable.

43

Q Why do some teenagers get pimples and others don't?

A The increase in hormones at puberty often causes increased oiliness and skin breakouts. The ovary and adrenal gland both produce significant amounts of male hormones (androgens), which stimulate glands in the skin. Some skin types are more susceptible to these hormonal changes. Bacteria may cause inflammation in skin pores that are clogged from the excess oil and secretions. As the reproductive hormones become more regulated, acne usually improves. However, some women are prone to acne their entire lives.

44

Q What medications best control acne?

A There are many over-the-counter and prescription medications available to treat acne. It's important to keep the skin clean with regular use of soap and water. Harsh or deodorant soaps should not be used. Cetaphil soap is a good choice. Over-the-counter drying agents such as Clearasil and Oxy are good. If more help is needed, a doctor can prescribe oral antibiotics or a topical application of a skin antibiotic such as Cleocin R (clindamycin). Careful application of retinoic acid decreases the blocked pores that lead to some acne formation. However, this medication can cause significant skin peeling and makes the skin sun sensitive. Birth control pills are also helpful because they even out hormone fluctuations and decrease the production of male hormones.

45

Q What should you tell a teenager about the dangers of sun damage?

A Telling a teenager that tanning booths and sunbathing are going to increase her chances of cancer and wrinkles doesn't usually make much of an impression. One severe sunburn markedly increases the risk of malignant melanoma, a skin cancer that can be fatal. Emphasize this risk. Provide her with a sunscreen that has at least an spf 15 and a fragrance and feel she likes. Shop with her for a cool hat or T-shirt she can use to protect herself from long days at the pool or beach.

46

Q Is there a makeup with sunblock that should be used for protection?

A There are foundations with built-in sunscreens. A water-based foundation, without moisturizer, is less likely to cause an acne flair up. The oil-based products can block pores, increasing acne and blackhead formation. Don't forget to put the foundation, or a lotion with sunscreen, on the neck also. The product should have an spf 15 or higher sunscreen.

47

Q At what age should a parent be concerned about her daughter's teeth being crooked?

A Children should begin having regular dental checkups at the age of three or four. The dentist will refer a patient to an orthodontist if correction of crooked or misaligned teeth is necessary.

48

Q What can a teenager do about strong body odor?

A The increase in sex hormones during puberty stimulates the sweat and sebaceous glands under the arms (axilla) and in the groin region, which increases body odor. Daily showers or bathing with a mild soap and water are usually adequate to control odor. An underarm deodorant can be introduced to help with the odor between washings.

49

Q When should a parent be concerned about a teenage girl staying in her room and not wanting to be with the family?

A Teenagers are moody and will spend time in their rooms listening to music, watching television, and talking to friends on the phone. They should be given a certain amount of privacy and respect for their property. Friends become increasingly more important than family. The teenager needs the time alone to help her move from dependent child to independent young person. Falling grades in school and increased isolation can be a warning sign for depression or substance abuse. If you have any concerns or questions, contact your physician or a professional counselor. Don't let problems simmer. Proactive intervention can be critical.

50

Q What should you do if one of your daughter's friends is making herself vomit after meals?

A Eating disorders such as bulimia and anorexia nervosa are encouraged by our society's focus on being thin. The bulimic often gorges herself with food and then induces vomiting. The use of laxatives, diuretics, and excessive exercise is also common. The young woman with anorexia nervosa is usually very thin but sees herself as fat. Her body image is distorted, and she cannot see what she looks like in the mirror or to another person. These disorders are serious and can be life threatening. Parents who suspect an eating disorder should reach out for medical help and professional counseling. Your daughter can suggest her friend tell her parents or look in the phone book for Overeaters Anonymous or ANAD, twelve-step programs focused on all types of eating disorders.

51

Q What is the best thing to say to a teenage girl who has decided growing up means smoking with her friends?

A Puberty and adolescence is a difficult time. A great deal of experimenting goes on to help teens develop their own code of ethics and morals. It is important to show them healthy adult behaviors. Discussions about addictions can be carefully woven into discussions about television shows, movies, or other things that interest teenagers. Consult a physician for pamphlets or literature you can give her to read.

Menstruation

52

Q What's happening to a woman when she feels like she's going crazy the week before her menstrual cycle?

A Many women experience mood changes a few days to two weeks before their period while others have none of the symptoms of premenstrual syndrome (PMS). Irritability, anxiety, depression, trouble sleeping, and a bloated feeling are some complaints physicians hear from patients. Most physicians now agree that PMS has a physiological basis.

53

Q How is premenstrual syndrome diagnosed?

A The diagnosis of PMS is a clinical one based on the exclusion of other problems that can cause the same symptoms. Women who have a biochemical depression can have an increase or exacerbation of symptoms prior to their period. Many other problems can mimic PMS including low thyroid. A physician can rule out causes other than PMS by taking a careful history, physical exam, blood tests, and examining a diary a woman has kept for several cycles noting her behaviors and the foods she's eaten.

54

Q Is there anything that can relieve PMS symptoms?

A PMS can be successfully treated once an accurate diagnosis is made. Lifestyle changes are the first line of therapy. Although PMS is not due to a vitamin deficiency, living on donuts, coffee, and diet drinks can certainly make symptoms worse. Eating a healthy diet, exercising regularly, getting enough sleep, and keeping stress to a minimum are important.

55

Q Are there any medications that can be prescribed to help with PMS?

A First, you should make sure that you and your physician have spent the time necessary to be certain of the diagnosis of PMS before starting any medical therapy. In addition, be sure that you have initiated lifestyle modifications, such as stress-reduction techniques, regular exercise, and good nutrition, to help manage the symptoms of PMS. Women with moderate to severe PMS (only about 5 percent of all women) often need medication to help control their symptoms. There are two classes of medication that have been shown to significantly help PMS: antidepressants and antianxiety medications. Prozac has been the most-studied antidepressant in the therapy of PMS. Sometimes even low doses of Prozac, such as 10 mg daily, can help. Other antidepressants, such as Zoloft and Paxil, may also be effective. Remember that these medications are not addictive and have relatively few side effects.

The antianxiety drug Xanax (alprazolam) is also effective for the treatment of PMS, especially in women whose main complaint is anxiety or irritability. This medication has a high addiction potential and must be carefully monitored. It should be given only during the specific time of symptoms and then gradually tapered off after the start of menses. Sudden withdrawal without tapering the dose can cause many symptoms. Buspar, which also treats anxiety but is not addictive, is helpful for some women with recurring premenstrual anxiety.

56

Q How do alternative techniques like yoga, acupuncture, and exercise help relieve symptoms of PMS?

A Any technique that decreases stress often helps with PMS symptoms. PMS in addition to other life pressures can equal stress overload. Yoga, tai chi, meditation, acupuncture, and exercise can all decrease your response to stress and therefore improve the symptoms you experience.

57

Q What happens during a menstrual period?

A The menstrual cycle starts with the onset of vaginal bleeding. Since a pregnancy didn't occur, the uterine lining is being cleared to prepare for the next chance of conception. A mature egg is released from the ovary usually in about the middle of the cycle. During egg development, estrogen is produced from the ovary, which causes growth of the lining of the uterus (endometrium). After egg release, both estrogen and progesterone are

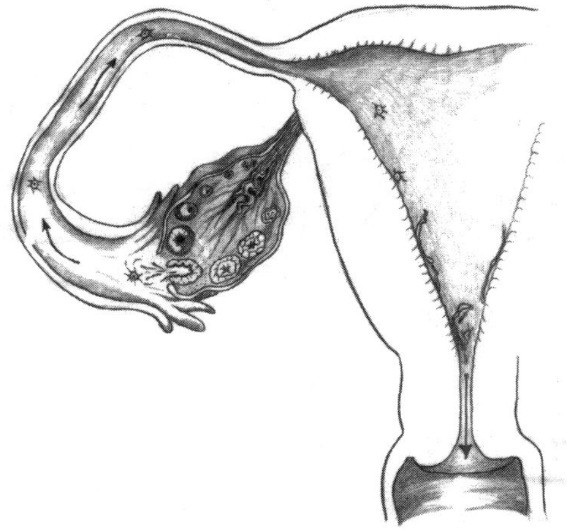

produced by the ovary. These hormones prepare the uterus for implantation of an embryo. If pregnancy doesn't occur, the uterine lining has sloughed off again, starting a new cycle.

58

Q How can a woman tell if she's ovulating?

A When the egg is mature, there is a sudden rise and then a fall in estrogen that causes the release of LH, a hormone from the anterior pituitary gland at the base of the brain. LH produces enzymes in the wall of the follicle which dissolve or weaken it. As the wall gets thinner, the pressure of the fluid in the follicle causes it to rupture, releasing the egg. The LH surge begins about thirty-six to forty hours prior to egg release and peaks about twenty-four hours before ovulation. Since this hormone is water soluble, LH levels can be measured in the urine. This is the basis of the home test kits used to detect impending ovulation. Regular monthly cycles usually indicate regular ovulation.

59

Q How can a woman tell if she's pregnant?

A If conception has taken place, the embryo, which is implanting in the uterine wall, produces a new hormone called HCG (human chorionic gonadotropin). This pregnancy hormone stimulates continued estrogen and progesterone production by the ovaries. Therefore, the start of a new period is prevented. Modern pregnancy tests are based on the measurement of HCG in urine or blood.

60

Q Why do some women have severe menstrual cramps and others don't?

A Menstrual cramps, technically termed dysmenorrhea, are physical symptoms caused by the contraction of the uterine wall. There is an increased pressure caused by the contraction of the smooth muscle that forms the wall of the uterus. The uterine lining breaks down during menses and releases a group of chemicals called prostaglandins, which cause the muscle contractions. The same compounds can stimulate contractions of the gastrointestinal tract causing increased numbers of bowel movements, diarrhea, and nausea.

61

Q Is there something wrong with a woman who is so irregular she never knows when she is going to get her period?

A Most women have a menstrual period every twenty-six to thirty-two days. A significant number of women, even after the completion of puberty, continue to have irregular cycles sometimes skipping one or more months. Their cycles are irregular because egg release or ovulation is irregular. The most common cause of irregular cycles is a hormone imbalance called polycystic ovarian disease (PCO), sometimes called Stein-Leventhal syndrome. These women have plenty of estrogen but fail to ovulate. The eggs (follicles) try to develop in the ovary but can't mature enough to be released. Therefore they hover around the edges of the ovaries and become small cysts. The ovaries and sometimes the adrenal glands can produce excess amounts of male hormone (androgens), which cause some women with PCO to experience abnormal hair growth on the face (hirsutism), oily skin, acne, and increased body weight. The irregular ovulation can be treated with the use of birth control pills, which also suppresses many of the other symptoms. If pregnancy is desired, clomiphene, "the fertility pill," usually induces ovulation.

62

Q Would a doctor ever recommend surgery for menstrual problems?

A Although many menstrual problems can be adequately treated with education and medications, sometimes surgical therapy is necessary. Uterine fibroids can cause excessive bleeding and may require removal through surgery. Some women delay medical evaluation so long that they have a low blood count (anemia) and medications may not control the bleeding quickly enough. In this situation, a dilation and curettage (D and C) may be necessary. Most D and Cs can be avoided if the patient seeks medical help early. Some women have heavy or irregular bleeding that can't be controlled by medications or a conservative surgical procedure. A hysterectomy may be necessary if other methods of control do not work.

63

Q What is a D and C?

A A D and C or dilation and curettage is a common procedure used to clean out the inside of the uterus. As with all surgeries, there are risks. During the procedure, the patient is usually given a sedative medication through an IV so she falls asleep. The inside of the vagina is cleansed with an antiseptic solution and the mouth of the uterus (cervix) is dilated to allow instruments to be placed inside the uterine cavity. Sometimes a gentle suction device is used to remove excess uterine lining or pregnancy tissue. A woman usually experiences a little cramping discomfort when she wakes up but recovers rapidly.

64

Q What type of procedure done for excessive bleeding doesn't require an incision?

A A relatively new procedure called endometrial ablation can be used to control abnormal bleeding that isn't associated with cancer or premalignant changes. Endometrial ablation is usually done as an outpatient procedure. No incision is necessary. The cervix is dilated to allow passage of a laser probe or a roller ball, which applies electrical energy to literally "burn out" the uterine lining (endometrium). Like all surgical procedures, endometrial ablation carries the risk of complication such as damage to the bladder, rectum, or abdominal organs as well as excessive bleeding or infection. However, most patients recover quickly and return to their normal schedules within several days. Some women avoid a hysterectomy by having this type of surgery.

65

Q What would cause a woman to bleed so heavily she can't even leave the house?

A Heavy menstrual periods are most often caused by a hormone imbalance, which can be controlled with medication. However, uterine fibroids, polyps, miscarriage or a problem with a pregnancy, and cancer can also cause the excessive flow. A women can become severely anemic from the recurrent heavy blood loss. If you've been bleeding this heavily, go to the doctor for an evaluation. Treated early, most problems can be controlled or corrected.

66

Q What is a fibroid tumor?

A A fibroid is a benign smooth muscle tumor that is most commonly found in the uterus. Although unusual, they can be found in the smooth muscle of the gastrointestinal (GI) tract such as the esophagus, stomach, or intestines. It is rare for these lesions to have any malignant potential. These benign tumors can become very large and cause pain and heavy bleeding. Fibroids found in the uterus are sometimes called myomas and can be underneath the uterine lining (submucosal). They can also be in the wall of the uterus (intramural) or project out from the surface of the uterus (subserosal). The submucosal fibroids are most likely to cause abnormal bleeding. Fibroids are common and are often asymptomatic. Just because a woman has an asymptomatic fibroid doesn't mean that she needs to have anything done. There are medications that temporarily decrease the size of the fibroid. If a surgical approach is necessary, a myomectomy may be performed to remove the fibroids and reconstruct the uterus or the entire uterus may be removed in a hysterectomy. Because this is a major surgery, it should be done by an experienced gynecologist.

67

Q What are polyps?

A Polyps are benign, fingerlike growths that most often occur on the inside of the uterus (endometrium) or the cervix. If a cervical polyp is identified at the time of a pelvic examination, the clinician can often remove it at that time. Most women complain of a mild cramp when a polyp is removed. Stitches aren't usually needed. A hysteroscopy or D and C are needed to remove polyps inside the uterus.

68

Q Is it okay for a woman to use tampons if she's never had sex?

A Most women who have never had intercourse have no difficulty using tampons. The opening of the virginal vagina (introitus) is usually adequate for the insertion of even a supersized tampon. These tissues stretch and are pliable. Since inserting a tampon is a learned skill, it is important to read the package directions carefully prior to insertion. Try a small or junior tampon first with a thin coating of petroleum jelly to make insertion easy. Gentle pressure usually separates the walls to easily admit the applicator of the tampon. In rare cases, some women have a thick covering or hymen over all or most of the opening of the vagina. The covering has to be surgically removed if it blocks the menstrual flow from the vagina. The use of a tampon is a personal decision and should not be based on virginity. If there is a problem with insertion, consult a health-care provider for help.

69

Q How should a woman decide whether to use a tampon or a sanitary pad?

A Use of tampons or pads is a matter of personal choice, comfort, and activity. The tampon may be more convenient if you're active in sports. Tampons make it possible to participate in water sports even during heavy menses. There is no objectionable odor from tampons since most odor doesn't occur until the menstrual flow comes in contact with air. Therefore, there is no benefit to using deodorant tampons. Some women prefer the sanitary pads that have improved in design and comfort over the past few years.

70

Q What is toxic shock syndrome?

A This condition is caused by the production of a toxin by certain types of staph bacteria. It is important to always wash your hands prior to insertion and removal of a tampon, change the tampon at least three times a day, use the smallest tampon that is adequate for your menstrual flow, and call a physician immediately if you experience high fever with a rash during your menstrual period.

71

Q Should a woman be concerned about not having periods for months at a time if she exercises a lot and has very little body fat?

A Most women have a menstrual period every twenty-six to thirty-two days. The absence of a menstrual cycle is called amenorrhea. Absence of menstrual cycles is likely to occur in women who have low estrogen levels. The low levels may in fact be due to low body weight or elevated prolactin. Prolactin is normally elevated when a woman is pregnant or breastfeeding. However, abnormal prolactin production can be an indication of a serious problem, such as a tumor near the anterior pituitary gland. Consult your doctor for an evaluation if you have inappropriate milk in your breasts. Low estrogen levels increase the risk of early or premature bone thinning or osteoporosis. Often female athletes think exercise will prevent osteoporosis when, in fact, exercising in excess can cause low estrogen and resulting bone loss. It is important to consult your physician for a personal assessment.

72

Q Can a woman have intercourse during her period?

A Many traditional cultures such as the Hebrews have forbidden women to have intercourse during their menstrual flow. The women were seen as "unclean." Most health-care specialists don't think there is any medical reason not to have sex during your period. Some physicians do point out that sexually transmitted diseases such as gonorrhea are more likely to be transmitted during menstrual flow. Others think that intercourse during menses might increase the risk of women developing endometriosis. There are no clear medical contraindications to sex during menses. It is a personal choice.

Pregnancy

73

Q Why would a doctor say someone is six weeks pregnant when the woman knows she is four weeks?

A Pregnancy is counted from the first day of the last menstrual period. Therefore, the two weeks of the conception cycle when a woman is not pregnant are included in the pregnancy date.

74

Q What exactly is an ectopic pregnancy?

A The sperm and egg join (fertilization) in an area of the Fallopian tube called the ampulla. After staying in the tube and dividing for several days, the embryo moves down to enter the uterine cavity. Sometimes the embryo fails to move down the tube into the uterus. The embryo begins to grow in the tube instead of in the uterus, creating an ectopic (or tubal) pregnancy. Left untreated, the tube will sometimes rupture, causing massive internal bleeding and endangering the life of the mother. Sometimes the tube has to be removed.

75

Q What are the risk factors for developing an ectopic pregnancy?

A Some women with seemingly normal tubes can experience an ectopic pregnancy. However, this is more likely to occur if the tube has been damaged by a previous infection or endometriosis. Therefore, patients with a history of a prior ectopic pregnancy, tubal surgery, or a pelvic infection are at high risk.

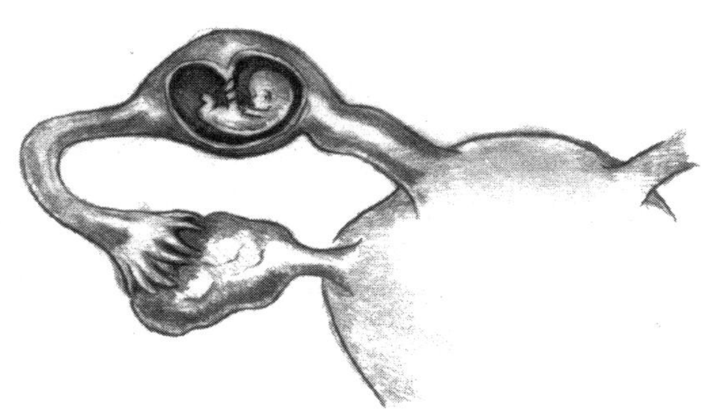

76

Q How are ectopic pregnancies diagnosed?

A Before ultrasound, ectopic pregnancies were usually diagnosed in the emergency room when the patient was admitted with severe abdominal pain and internal blood loss. Today, most ectopic pregnancies are diagnosed before a rupture by a health-care provider using vaginal ultrasound.

77

Q What are the treatment options for a woman with an ectopic pregnancy?

A There is still no way to save the embryo when a woman is treated for an ectopic pregnancy. It must be removed surgically or destroyed with medication. One way to treat an ectopic pregnancy is to perform a laparoscopy. An incision is made over the ectopic pregnancy in the Fallopian tube and the pregnancy tissue is removed. Any bleeding is carefully controlled, and the tube is allowed to heal on its own. The amount of pregnancy hormone in the woman's blood is carefully followed until it is zero to ensure that all of the pregnancy tissue was removed. Another treatment is to give the patient a chemotherapy drug called methotrexate. Often one dose of this medication will cause resorption of the ectopic pregnancy. Although the drug has potentially serious side effects including low blood count, loss of hair, and ulceration of the GI tract, a one-time dose is usually without serious side effects.

78

Q Can a woman with one fetus lodged in a tube have it removed and remain pregnant with another fetus that is correctly placed?

A It is common for a woman using fertility drugs to release more than one egg. Removing the ectopic pregnancy through laparoscopy (LSC) doesn't harm the normally developing embryo in the uterus.

79

Q Are fetal reductions safe?

A Because of the use of fertility medications and in vitro fertilization techniques, multiple fetuses are frequently being conceived. The more babies that occupy the uterus, the greater the chance of significant prematurity and serious illness or death for the fetuses. Some couples decide to have one or more fetuses removed to protect the others. This procedure is done with ultrasound guidance.

80

Q What are the chances of having a healthy pregnancy after a Fallopian tube has been removed?

A A woman has an excellent chance of pregnancy if she has one healthy tube and a normal ovary on the same side. Although it may take longer than average to achieve a pregnancy with two ovaries and only one tube, you should be successful over time. In most women, each ovary ovulates about half the time. Therefore, one-half the total number of ovulations will be from the ovary that doesn't have a tube near it. She should have a normal chance of pregnancy when she ovulates on the side with her remaining tube. If a tube was removed because of an ectopic pregnancy, there is risk for a second such experience.

81

Q What causes a woman to have a miscarriage?

A Most spontaneous early pregnancy losses are due to an abnormal embryo. A genetic mistake occurs during egg or sperm production, when the sperm and egg merge, or in the first divisions of the embryo. These are random genetic mistakes. The abnormal embryos do not survive, and the woman will have a miscarriage. There are other causes of early pregnancy loss, such as inadequate production of progesterone after ovulation. If sufficient progesterone isn't produced, the uterine lining (endometrium) will not be adequately prepared for embryo attachment. Sometimes uterine fibroids can distort the uterine cavity or decrease the blood supply to the uterus, causing a miscarriage.

Some parents carry an abnormal chromosome that causes recurrent genetic abnormalities in their embryos, resulting in multiple miscarriages. Infections such as toxoplasmosis and an organism called mycoplasma are responsible for some pregnancy losses. Fertility specialists have recently identified immunological problems, such as lupus antibodies, that cause multiple miscarriages. If a woman loses two or more pregnancies without delivering a healthy baby, her physician will likely recommend additional testing for these types of problems.

82

Q Is a woman able to have a baby after a miscarriage?

A Miscarriages are common. A physician will not usually recommend a medical evaluation unless there have been at least two miscarriages without a normal pregnancy. Three miscarriages without a normal pregnancy is technically termed recurrent spontaneous abortion, or recurrent early pregnancy loss. Most women who have a miscarriage are able to experience normal pregnancies.

83

Q Can miscarriages be prevented?

A There is no known treatment for the risk of spontaneous, random, genetic abnormalities, which are common in human pregnancy and cause pregnancy loss. However, there may be recurrent causes of miscarriages that can be identified and treated. For example, a culture can be done of the cervix to see if an infection may be causing pregnancy loss, or an antibiotic such as doxycycline may be prescribed. Certain other infections, such as cytomegalovirus and toxoplasmosis, which are typically diagnosed by a blood test, can cause miscarriage but will not cause recurrent pregnancy loss. One of the most common causes of miscarriage, which can be treated with medication, is low progesterone production. An Xray of the uterus, called a hysterosalpingogram, can determine if a fibroid or uterine septum might be distorting the shape of the uterine cavity. Surgical therapy can remove a mass or septum. Some women produce antibodies that are associated with the autoimmune disease lupus and can cause miscarriage. A laboratory study can be done to measure these antibodies. In rare instances, adults can have a genetic abnormality that causes recurrent pregnancy loss. What this means is that the adult appears normal, but a piece of one chromosome is "stuck on" another chromosome. The resulting eggs or sperm can then be genetically imbalanced. A chromosomal analysis of the male and female partners can identify this as the cause of recurrent pregnancy loss. If any of these factors are found, a reproductive endocrinologist should be consulted.

84

Q What is Down's syndrome?

A A genetic mistake may occur during egg or sperm production, when the sperm and egg merge, or in the first divisions of the embryo. When an extra chromosome 21 gets into an embryo, Down's syndrome will occur. Children with Down's syndrome are mentally challenged and can have a variety of physical handicaps. This disorder can be diagnosed prenatally by a genetic amniocentesis. Families with one child with Down's syndrome are at risk for a second, and they should seek genetic counseling.

85

Q Is it possible to increase the chances of conceiving a male or female child?

A The sex of a baby is determined by the type of sperm which fertilizes the egg. The male-producing sperm are slightly lighter than the female-producing sperm, and there are separation techniques such as centrifugation which can increase the percentage of male-producing sperm in semen. The enriched part of the semen specimen can then be used for artificial insemination. However, there is some uncertainty among physicians about how much the chance of a male birth can be increased using these techniques. Improving the chance of a female birth is even more difficult. In the near future, using in vitro fertilization, sex selection may be routinely available.

Over-the-counter kits which claim to be able to provide sex selection at home using natural intercourse are not very effective, even though they are successful about 50 percent of the time! Most couples just decide to go ahead with natural conception and let chance decide the sex of their offspring.

86

Q Will a previous pelvic infection affect a woman's ability to get pregnant?

A The type and severity of the infection are important in determining your risk of permanent damage from the infection. About 12 percent of women will have severely damaged or blocked tubes after experiencing pelvic inflammatory disease (PID) with a high fever and pain. Each subsequent episode of infection increases the risk of tubal closure. A pelvic infection also increases the risk of an ectopic pregnancy. If you are pregnant and have had an infection or prior ectopic pregnancy, be sure to see your physician early to test your hormone levels and get at least one early ultrasound at six or six and a half weeks to be certain the pregnancy is progressing normally.

87

Q Can a fibroid on the uterus affect a woman's chances of becoming pregnant or cause complications during a pregnancy?

A Most women with fibroids don't have any trouble getting or staying pregnant. Occasionally a fibroid distorts the inside of the uterus enough that implantation is unlikely. These submucosal fibroids can often be removed by an outpatient surgical procedure using a hysteroscope. Sometimes fibroids become so big that they impede the normal blood supply to the uterus, which can cause problems with pregnancy. If the uterus is about the size of a three-month pregnancy, due to fibroids, a myomectomy may need to be done to remove the fibroids but preserve the uterus for pregnancy. Because of their location, these benign, smooth muscle tumors can block one or both Fallopian tubes. There is also a rare risk of cancer, so a fibroid should be removed if it shows rapid growth. A cesarean section may be needed if the fibroids grow during pregnancy in an area that prevents a normal vaginal birth.

88

Q How can a woman tell when she's fertile if she has irregular menstrual cycles?

A A woman with markedly irregular menses, every four to twelve weeks, should consider seeing a physician who can prescribe medication to regulate ovulation. Your chance for a successful pregnancy is dependent on ovulation. If a woman's menstrual cycle occurs every four to six weeks, a home LH test kit may be helpful in detecting ovulation.

89

Q How can a woman increase her chances of becoming pregnant?

A If you are normally fertile, you can increase your chance of conception by optimum timing of intercourse. Purchase an LH surge test kit; Ovuquick or Clear Plan Easy are good choices. These home test kits are able to detect the surge in urine of the hormone that actually causes release of the egg. Be certain to follow the instructions carefully. The test will turn positive at the peak of the LH surge. Egg release occurs about twenty-four hours after the peak of LH. If you have intercourse the day of the LH surge, this is optimum timing for pregnancy. It is better to be a little early than too late. Sperm can live for twenty-four to seventy-two hours. To determine your average day of ovulation, start to keep a menstrual cycle calendar. Ovulation occurs about fourteen days prior to the start of a period.

90

Q What are the best steps to take to decrease the chance of having a baby with a birth defect?

A We don't know what causes many birth defects. It is good to discuss any history of birth defects in your family with your physician prior to pregnancy. Some birth defects run in families. If this is true of your family or your husband's, your physician may suggest that you have an amniocentesis when you become pregnant. Some birth defects are caused by infections. Have your blood checked prior to becoming pregnant to see if you are immune to rubella (German measles) and chicken pox. Do not drink alcohol, use tobacco, or use recreational drugs (such as marijuana, cocaine, heroine, amphetamines), diet pills, herb preparations from the health food store, and megavitamins, especially vitamin A or beta carotene. Don't take any medication while you're trying to get pregnant that isn't approved by your physician. Start taking a prenatal vitamin with folic acid before pregnancy. Eat fresh fruits and vegetables and get your nutrients from a healthy diet. Although there is no scientific data pointing to the dangers of environmental toxins, it is recommended to avoid pesticides, paint fumes, and hair permanents.

91

Q How old is too old to have a baby?

A Although the best time to have your children physiologically and genetically is in your late teens and early twenties, many women in their forties are now choosing to have children with their own eggs or with egg donations from younger women. When to have a baby is a personal decision that a woman must make herself after talking to her doctor and weighing the possible medical risks to herself and her baby. Potential parents should also consider the needs of their future offspring when evaluating their desires.

92

Q Can a woman who has had a tubal ligation get pregnant?

A We always encourage patients to consider a tubal ligation as a permanent procedure. However, there are two successful ways to achieve pregnancy after a tubal is performed. The tubes can be reconnected by a major microsurgical procedure if there is enough healthy tube remaining. A uterine X ray (hysterosalpingogram HSG) needs to be done to determine how much healthy tube is left attached to the uterus. A laparoscopy (LSC) is also necessary to evaluate how much tube is left on the distal segment, which is the part nearest the ovary. Some forms of tubal ligation are more successfully reversed than others. If a tubal reversal is not possible, in vitro fertilization can be performed. Since the egg is removed from the ovary, incubated with sperm for fertilization, and then placed into the uterine cavity during the in vitro process, Fallopian tubes are not needed for conception.

93

Q Does a low sperm count mean a man will never be able to get his wife pregnant?

A Inseminations are a generally safe and relatively inexpensive way to improve the chances of pregnancy for some men with a low sperm count. The procedure begins by collecting sperm through masturbation or a special condom. The sperm are separated from the natural fluid around them, the seminal fluid, and resuspended in a nutrient fluid in the physician's office. This fluid containing the sperm is placed in a small flexible tube, which is threaded through the cervix. Most women say the catheter placement feels like a Pap smear. The sperm are then injected directly into the uterine cavity. They still have to swim out the uterus into the Fallopian tubes to meet the egg, but this technique eliminates the possibility that any sperm will be lost in the folds of the vagina, which is common during intercourse. If this technique works, it is much less expensive and less stressful than in vitro fertilization. If in vitro fertilization is necessary, the sperm and the eggs can be placed together in a culture dish or the sperm can be inserted into the eggs through a process called ICSI (intracytoplasmic sperm insertion).

94

Q How long should a couple expect it to take them to get pregnant after they stop using birth control?

A Studies have shown that eight out of ten healthy young couples will be pregnant in one year of unprotected intercourse. More than 90 percent will be pregnant in two years. Although these statistics indicate that there may be a fertility problem if you haven't gotten pregnant within two years of unprotected sex, this isn't always true. Fertility starts to fall quickly about the age of thirty-eight. A woman under thirty-five should wait for a full year of unprotected intercourse before she starts a fertility evaluation. A woman near or over forty should consider starting fertility therapy with a reproductive endocrinologist if she doesn't become pregnant in six months of unprotected intercourse. A reproductive endocrinologist is an OB/GYN physician who has done a two-year fellowship specializing in hormonal disorders and fertility.

95

Q What are the options for a single woman who wants to adopt a child?

A More and more single women are adopting children. The chances of adoption increase if you are interested in a non-Caucasian child. RESOLVE is a self-help infertility organization that offers excellent adoption resource information. Network with others who have completed a successful foreign adoption to learn how that process works as well.

96

Q What is in vitro fertilization?

A In vitro literally means "in glass." In this procedure, the female takes injectable medications that stimulate the production of multiple eggs. When the eggs are mature, as determined by ultrasound and hormone levels, they are removed using a needle attached to a vaginal ultrasound transducer. While the ovary is being watched on an ultrasound, the needle is advanced through the vaginal wall into the individual follicles (egg units) in the ovaries. The eggs are removed by suction and taken to the laboratory. The woman receives some form of anesthesia or pain medication during the egg recovery. The husband's sperm are placed into the culture dishes with the eggs. Usually natural fertilization occurs. Sometimes fertilization may be assisted by direct sperm injection. If fertilization is successful, the embryo is observed for normal growth. It is placed through the cervix forty-eight to seventy-two hours after egg retrieval. Progesterone is usually given to prepare the uterine lining for embryo implantation.

97

Q When is in vitro fertilization usually recommended?

A Initially in vitro was used to help women with tubal blockage or severe pelvic adhesions become pregnant. Now it's also being used to treat male infertility. As the success rates have increased and more sophisticated aids to fertilization have been developed, more and more couples are choosing this option. A single in vitro cycle may cost between seventy-five hundred and twelve thousand dollars, and there are no guarantees of success with this procedure.

98

Q Will a lubricant used for intercourse interfere with a woman's ability to get pregnant?

A Although sexual lubricants are not reliable forms of contraception, they may decrease the chance of pregnancy. Baby oil, petroleum jelly (such as Vaseline), and other oils make it difficult for sperm to swim into the cervix. Even water-based lubricants such as K-Y Jelly and Astroglide are believed to impede sperm motility. It is best to avoid any vaginal products while you are fertile if you wish to conceive.

99

Q Is severe pain in the right lower part of my abdomen during a pregnancy serious?

A This discomfort may be as serious as an ectopic pregnancy, which is potentially life threatening, or it may be as simple as round ligament syndrome. A woman who has round ligament syndrome will experience a feeling like a muscle spasm in the ligament that attaches the uterus to the pubic bone. It can be quite painful but only lasts a short time. Any woman experiencing persistent abdominal pain during pregnancy should consult her doctor.

100

Q How could a woman be carrying a baby in her abdomen?

A An abdominal pregnancy is a rare and serious complication of pregnancy. The egg and sperm meet normally in the Fallopian tube and fertilization takes place. In an abdominal pregnancy, instead of going down the tube to the uterine cavity (the womb), the embryo goes into the abdominal cavity through the opening of the tube and attaches to the bowel or liver. As the placenta grows, it attaches to other areas often causing pain. In extremely rare instances these babies are carried to term, but more often, the pregnancy must be terminated to protect the health of the mother. The doctor can't remove the placenta at surgery because it is attached to so many organs that uncontrolled bleeding would occur. The umbilical cord is tied and cut to remove the fetus, and the placenta is left in place. The mother is given a chemotherapy drug called methotrexate to cause the placenta to be reabsorbed by the body.

101

Q Why in the world would a woman be eating laundry starch?

A Some women, who are iron deficient, crave laundry starch or certain types of clay or ice. This type of eating activity is called pica. The substances are not usually dangerous when consumed, but they do keep the woman from making better, healthy diet choices. Pica is most common during pregnancy and in certain cultural communities. Treatment is based on education, iron supplements, and a healthy diet plan.

102

Q What is an amniocentesis?

A This is a test that takes a small portion of amniotic fluid, which contains living fetal cells, from the uterine cavity of a pregnant woman. The cells can be grown in culture to evaluate the chromosomes, and specific substances can be measured from the fluid to detect abnormalities and general health of the baby.

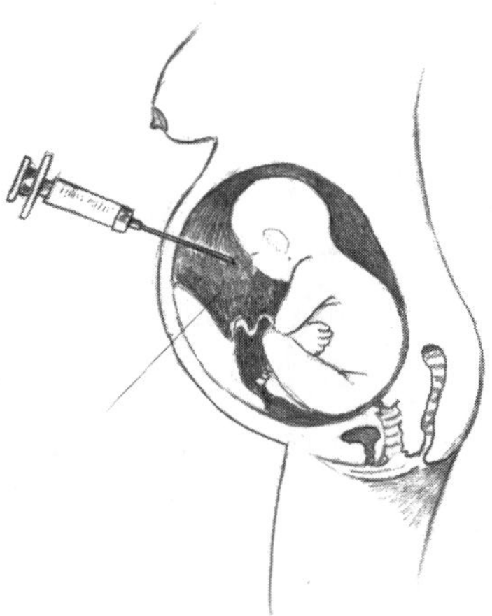

103

Q Why would a woman have an amniocentesis?

A Couples who have a family history of birth defects or other genetic diseases may want to have information on their baby before its birth. In addition, any abnormal ultrasound or level of alpha-fetoprotein in the woman's blood during pregnancy would indicate the test should be done. The American College of Obstetrics and Gynecology recommends that amniocentesis be offered to every woman thirty-five and older because the incidence of birth defects, especially Down's syndrome, increases with the age of the mother.

104

Q What does an amniocentesis say about the health of the fetus?

A Genetic defects such as Down's syndrome can be detected by evaluating the fetal chromosomes. In addition, tests will indicate if a fetus might have a neurological abnormality where the central nervous system (brain and spinal cord) wasn't formed normally. At times, the procedure is done to determine whether the baby would be able to breathe on its own if delivery was necessary.

105

Q What are the risks of amniocentesis?

A Amniocentesis is a fairly safe procedure. About one in two hundred procedures could cause a miscarriage. There is also the possibility that infection could be introduced into the uterus or the needle might cause damage to the fetus.

106

Q Why do doctors perform alpha-fetoprotein tests during pregnancy?

A This simple blood test screens for a number of birth abnormalities including neural tube defects, which is a central nervous system disorder, and Down's syndrome. Some women with an abnormal alpha-fetoprotein have normal pregnancies. This test simply indicates that further evaluation including ultrasound and amniocentesis should be done.

5

Menopause

107

Q What is menopause?

A Technically, menopause has been reached when a mature woman hasn't had a menstrual period for one year. Menopause occurs because women run out of healthy eggs that can be developed and released from the ovaries. FSH (Follicle Stimulating Hormone) is low prior to the onset of menopausal transition. When estrogen production starts to fall, the anterior pituitary hormones, LH and FSH, start to increase to stimulate more estrogen production. A persistently elevated FSH is the best laboratory test to detect if a woman is near menopause.

108

Q Why do some women's periods change when they are too young to be going through menopause?

A Irregular cycles can be caused by a number of factors. One is premature menopause, which is defined as the cessation of menses prior to the age of forty. Other reasons for irregular cycles include improper secretion of prolactin, excessively low body weight, thyroid disorders, and polycystic ovaries. See your health-care provider for a personal evaluation if you begin experiencing irregular periods.

109

Q What is perimenopause?

A The perimenopause encompasses the transition phase from normal, cyclical menses until the cessation of menstrual cycles. This phase often lasts two to seven years. The ovaries are starting to have decreased hormone production. Egg release, and therefore menses, becomes erratic. This can be an aggravating time of life because there is no predictability to the menstrual periods. Some women complain of mood swings, which may be due to swings in hormone production. Hot flushes (also called hot flashes) and difficulty sleeping are characteristic of perimenopause. Estrogen supplementation often helps many of these symptoms.

110

Q Do mothers and daughters tend to have the same experience with menopause?

A There is a trend for mothers and daughters to have similar menopause experiences. However, a lot depends on how you choose to manage your menopause symptoms. Whether they take hormones or not, some women never experience any problems. Women who are carefully monitored and decide to take hormonereplacement therapy usually find these medicines helpful in alleviating symptoms. Women who choose to avoid hormone replacement during the height of their symptoms in perimenopause may find help from alternative therapies such as vitamins, herbs, and exercise. Estrogen supplementation and regulation of menstrual cycles with a form of progesterone is the most successful therapy.

111

Q Can a woman determine when she will most likely go through menopause?

A The average age of menopause may be fifty-one, but just like puberty every woman goes through the process, known as climacteric, at her own pace. It is normal to be menopausal as early as age forty or as late as sixty. There is a tendency to go through menopause like the other women in your family. In addition, the earlier you start your cycles the longer you have them. Remember that perimenopausal transition can begin two to seven years prior to actual menopause. Symptoms such as hot flushes are common and may start around age forty.

112

Q What should a woman do if she can't get a good night's sleep?

A Hot flushes, one of the symptoms of menopausal transition, is responsible for poor quality sleep. Many of the negative symptoms of menopause, such as irritability and moodiness, may be due to a sleep disorder caused by recurrent hot flushes. Some women will wake up every hour during the night with hot flushes during the peak of menopausal symptoms. As the flushes diminish, sleep will improve. There are several medications that can help control hot flushes. If you think you are losing sleep because of hot flushes, consult your health-care provider for an evaluation.

113

Q What's the difference between natural and surgical menopause?

A Natural menopause is usually a gradual process in which the ovaries produce less and less hormones over several years. Menstrual cycles become less frequent and eventually stop. Surgical menopause takes place when the ovaries are removed. In this case, a woman goes through the entire menopause process in one day. Women experience the symptoms such as hot flushes and vaginal dryness whether they've gone through natural or surgical menopause. The symptoms may even be more severe in the surgical menopause because of the sudden withdrawal of estrogen production.

114

Q What should a woman do if she's exhausted all the time and just doesn't feel well?

A A woman between forty and sixty tends to blame every physical problem on hormones. And sometimes it is hormones. But there are other factors that can cause loss of energy and general "blahs." If you still have a uterus and are having irregular cycles, it is highly likely that you are going through menopausal transition. It is even more difficult to detect perimenopause in a woman who has had a hysterectomy since there are no menstrual cycles. A blood FSH test right after the start of menses or randomly taken in a woman without a uterus is the best test to use for the onset of perimenopause. Sometimes it is necessary to do a second FSH to confirm the result two weeks later. Remember that FSH can also be elevated because you are about to ovulate. A thyroid imbalance can also produce these symptoms. Depression, sleep deprivation, a connective tissue disorder, excessive stress, chronic hepatitis, and many other problems can produce nonspecific symptoms such as fatigue. A complete evaluation of your medical status and your lifestyle may be in order.

115

Q What is a hot flush?

A A hot flush, also referred to as a hot flash, is one of the most incapacitating symptoms of the transition phase to menopause. Generally, the sensation of heat starts in the chest or neck and spreads outward. A neuronal discharge from the brain starts the hot flush. The blood vessels of the skin are dilated even though the internal or core temperature of the body is normal. The woman's skin looks red and profuse sweating may occur. Often the heart rate increases, causing palpitations and a sensation that the heart is fluttering. Because of the shunting of blood to the skin and evaporative cooling from sweating, the woman may feel cold after the sensation of heat passes.

116

Q Is there anything that can be done to alleviate hot flushes?

A The most effective treatment for hot flushes is estrogen replacement. The frequency of hot flushes is increased by a warm, moist environment and stress. Adequate estrogen usually decreases the frequency and intensity of hot flushes. For women who can't take estrogen or whose hot flushes aren't adequately controlled by estrogen, an antihypertensive medication called clonidine directly inhibits hot flushes by suppressing the neuronal discharge from the brain. Clonidine, which is widely used in Europe, is available as a skin patch or an oral medication. Some women feel dizzy or faint when they use this medication and get up too fast from a sitting or lying position (orthostatic hypotension). The use of a synthetic progestin such as medroxyprogesterone acetate (Provera) by itself or in combination with estrogen also helps suppress hot flushes. For many, but not all women, hot flushes tend to decrease in frequency and intensity with age. They are usually worse in perimenopause and less frequent in postmenopause.

117

Q Why does the female body stop making estrogen?

A The majority of the natural estrogen is made in the ovaries by the developing egg units called follicles. Menopause occurs because we literally run out of good eggs. We receive all of the eggs we are ever going to have when we ourselves are embryos. The eggs are used up by ovulation and degeneration (atresia) over our reproductive lives. When the eggs are gone, estrogen production decreases. There is still the production of some weak estrogens. This happens by a bioconversion. The adrenal glands and ovaries both produce hormone precursors, which fat cells turn into weak estrogens. Thin women have less estrogen after menopause than overweight women. Therefore, osteoporosis and hot flushes are more common in women with low body fat.

118

Q Why do some doctors suggest taking hormones to help regulate cycles?

A Irregular cycles are caused by lack of regular egg release (ovulation). When estrogen is produced by a follicle that is trying to develop but fails to ovulate, progesterone is not produced in normal amounts. The uterine lining is stimulated to grow by the estrogen. However, the normal transformation of the cells does not occur due to progesterone deficiency. Estrogen and progesterone are out of balance. The best treatment is to supplement with a form of progesterone. The most commonly used medication is medroxyprogesterone acetate (Provera), which is a synthetic progestin. In addition to regulating the cycle, this hormone decreases the risk of uterine cancer. Most women who take this hormone can't even tell they are taking it, but some women get depressed or feel as if they have premenstrual syndrome. Natural oral micronized progesterone is another option. In addition, there are several low-dose birth control pills with only 20 mg of estrogen (Alesse or LoEstrin), which are very successful at regulating irregular cycles and are safe for low-risk women over thirty-five who don't smoke.

119

Q Why does one woman need estrogen when another woman of the same age doesn't?

A Keep in mind that there is a wide variation in timing for going through the process of menopause. Some women are menopausal at forty and others not until they are in their sixties. Perimenopause is a good time to start reading about the pros and cons of hormone-replacement therapy. Every woman needs to be well informed so that she can make an educated decision, as a partner with her physician, about hormone replacement.

120

Q What's the difference between a natural and synthetic estrogen?

A The estrogen used in birth control pills (ethinyl estradiol) is a synthetic form of estrogen; it is made in a laboratory.

Most of the estrogens used for menopausal hormone replacement are of natural origin. Premarin is a natural animal estrogen product purified from the urine of pregnant horses. Oral micronized estradiol (Estrace) is a natural plant product derived from wild Mexican yams.

121

Q What are the risks of taking estrogen?

A Although estrogen replacement has many health benefits, it does have some potential risks. If a woman who has a uterus takes estrogen without progesterone, she increases her risk of uterine cancer. However, if she balances the estrogen with a form of progesterone such as medroxyprogesterone acetate—5 mg for twelve days each month or 2.5 mg daily—she has no added risk of uterine cancer. In fact, she has a lower risk of uterine cancer than if she took no hormones at all.

It is also hotly debated whether estrogen supplementation after menopause increases the risk of breast cancer. Most of the studies that have looked at this issue have reported no association between breast cancer and estrogen replacement after menopause. However, several studies have suggested there is a significant risk, especially for long-term use.

There are many different types of estrogen: conjugated equine estrogen (Premarin), oral micronized estradiol (Estrace), estradiol by skin patch (Vivelle, Fempatch, Climana), estrogen injections, pellets, and gel. Studies are in progress to assess the risk of estrogen, but the final outcome will not be available until sometime in the twenty-first century.

122

Q What are the benefits of taking estrogen?

A There are many benefits to the short- and long-term use of estrogen replacement starting at the time of perimenopause. Estrogen relieves many of the symptoms associated with menopausal transition. It decreases the frequency and intensity of hot flushes and treats the vaginal atrophy (vaginal lining becomes thin and fragile without estrogen stimulation), which is associated with estrogen deprivation. Estrogen is also the most important factor in the prevention of osteoporosis. Studies strongly suggest that long-term estrogen replacement prevents 30 to 70 percent of heart disease. Estrogen increases the production of the "good" form of cholesterol, HDL. In addition, estrogen is a powerful antioxidant. It has a direct effect on blood vessels, making them less susceptible to damage. New information suggests that estrogen may play a part in the prevention of Alzheimer's disease, which is more common in women than men. It has been estimated by several studies that there is a 30 to 60 percent reduction in Alzheimer's with long-term estrogen replacement.

123

Q How does a woman decide if estrogen replacement is right for her?

A Every woman needs to assess the benefits and risks of estrogen for herself. First calculate your personal risk of osteoporosis, know your cholesterol profile, and assess your risks of heart disease and breast cancer. Schedule a discussion consultation with your health-care provider to help reach your final decision.

124

Q How does a woman know which type of estrogen is best for her?

A The most widely prescribed and best studied estrogen in the United States is conjugated equine estrogen (Premarin). It is an excellent product and offers all the potential benefits of estrogen therapy. However, there is no scientific evidence at this time to suggest that one type of oral estrogen is superior to another. Some women just seem to feel better on one or another.

The main estrogen produced in the ovaries prior to menopause is estradiol, making this form of estrogen seem more "natural." There is a conjugated oral estrogen (Ogen) and an oral micronized estrogen (estradiol, sold under the brand name Estrace), which are pure plant-derived estrogens. All of these estrogens are available as generic products. Since the estradiol is identical to the main ovarian estrogen, our traditional laboratory hormone assays are able to measure blood levels to detect adequate absorption. However, most women respond well to normal doses of estrogen and expensive blood studies are not usually needed.

125

Q How should a woman decide which method of taking estrogen she should use?

A There are different estrogen delivery systems, and all of them carry similar benefit-risk ratios. Oral estrogen offers perhaps more improvement in the cholesterol profile than the skin patch. This is because the oral estrogen travels through the gastrointestinal tract and then into the liver in its most concentrated form, improving the production of HDL (good) cholesterol. However, some prefer the skin patch because it delivers estrogen directly into the bloodstream, which is the way it is delivered from the ovaries naturally. If a woman has not had a hysterectomy, generally a form of progesterone must be added to the estrogen to prevent the increased risk of uterine cancer associated with unopposed estrogen. On the other hand, if a woman no longer has a uterus, pure estrogen, without progesterone, offers the best heart protection. Some have suggested that it is more natural to add progesterone to estrogen even if the woman has had a hysterectomy. I do not believe it is necessary to take progesterone if you aren't at risk for uterine cancer.

126

Q Does taking estrogen automatically lead to weight gain?

A Most women over fifty will gain three to five pounds a year unless they increase their regular exercise and maintain a healthy diet. A randomized medical research study was conducted with postmenopausal women in which half of them took .625 of conjugated estrogen and the other half took a placebo for one year. There was no significant difference between the two groups; both gained weight. A high dose of estrogen can increase fluid retention, but there is no evidence that the low dose of estrogen used during menopause will cause weight gain.

127

Q Is there a form of estrogen a vegetarian can take that's not from animal products?

A Two products, Estrace and Ogen, are made from wild Mexican yams. The estrogen in skin patches is also usually from plant products.

128

Q Does the same nausea that some women experience with birth control pills also occur with estrogen?

A Nausea is rare while taking hormone replacement because the estrogen dose is low compared to birth control pills. Keep in mind that you are replacing normal amounts of estrogen, the amount ovaries regularly produced, when you take climacteric hormone therapy.

129

Q What is progesterone?

A Progesterone is a natural hormone that is produced after egg release by the ovaries and in large amounts by the placenta during pregnancy. The main action of this hormone during the menstrual cycle is to prepare the uterine lining (endometrium) for implantation of a pregnancy. If a pregnancy doesn't occur, progesterone levels fall and menses begins. Adequate levels of progesterone oppose the actions of estrogen to help prevent uterine (endometrial) cancer. A synthetic or natural hormone that has progesterone-like activity is called a progestin.

130

Q Is there an alternative to taking a synthetic progesterone?

A Although the majority of women taking a synthetic progestin show no symptoms, there is a small number of women who become depressed, anxious, and irritable on this medication. The symptoms seem to be based on the dose being taken. Years ago, 10 mg of Provera a day was routinely prescribed to regulate menses and decrease the risk of uterine cancer. Today most women receive 5 mg for ten to fourteen days each month or 2.5 mg daily. Natural oral micronized progesterone is an alternative that rarely causes side effects, but it hasn't been as extensively studied as Provera. Because the natural hormone is metabolized faster than a synthetic, it should be taken twice daily: morning and night.

131

Q Are natural forms of hormones safer than synthetics?

A All hormones can cause complications and have potential benefits depending on the dosage, the length of time taken, and the other hormones or medicines used with it. Natural doesn't necessarily mean safe. Similarly, synthetic doesn't mean the hormone is bad or unsafe. Each has to be assessed on its own merits. Too much of any hormone can be dangerous.

132

Q Are there any herbal preparations, rather than medications from a physician, that help alleviate menopause symptoms?

A There is little scientific information about herbal preparations, which have been used by women in China, Japan, and other Eastern cultures for centuries. The U.S. government established the Office of Alternative Medicine at the National Institutes of Health in Washington, D.C., to study the potential benefits and risks of these types of products, which are not subject to the approval of the Food and Drug Administration. Hopefully we will know more about their safety and effectiveness in the near future.

133

Q Why do Asian women experience fewer problems with menopause than Caucasians?

A Western doctors are just beginning to look at the menopause experience in Eastern countries. It is possible that one reason these women experience fewer problems with menopause is cultural. For example, older women in Eastern societies are generally more respected and supported by their families as they age; they do not suffer from the negative connotation of aging that pervades Western cultures.

Medically speaking, their genetic makeup may allow them to respond differently to a decrease in estrogen product. The Eastern diet is high in soy products, which produce estrogen-like substances that suppress menopausal symptoms. For example, hot flushes are a relatively rare complaint of menopausal women in Eastern countries. There is also the possibility that the herbal remedies they use are controlling menopausal symptoms. Only recently have well-designed studies been organized by Western doctors to study the effects of various herbal remedies on menopause. We will have to wait for the results of these studies to find out which herbs really work and which are safe for use.

134

Q If menopause is a natural passage of life, why do we have to treat it like it's an illness?

A The average life expectancy of a woman in the 1900s was fifty, compared with eighty today. The medical field is beginning to understand the potential complications that can occur when a woman lives thirty or more years without estrogen. Menopause is not an illness but a phase of life with potential complications: osteoporosis, genital atrophy, and heart disease among them. Although not all women experience all of these complications, many of us face serious quality-of-life compromises without estrogen supplements. For example, osteoporosis, which can be warded off by estrogen supplements, can be deadly but is more likely to affect a woman's quality of life by forcing her to spend the last several years of her life in a nursing care facility. Women simply need to learn how to minimize the risks and optimize quality of life.

135

Q What treatments are available for fibroids?

A Fibroids are common, benign, smooth muscle tumors. Small fibroids that don't grow and cause symptoms don't require any treatment. Often fibroids become smaller after menopause. If fibroids become large or symptomatic, they can be removed by a surgery known as a myomectomy, which preserves the uterus. Depending on the size and location of the fibroids, a laparoscopy or hysteroscopy can be done on an outpatient basis. Some women opt to have a hysterectomy for fibroids if they don't want future pregnancies.

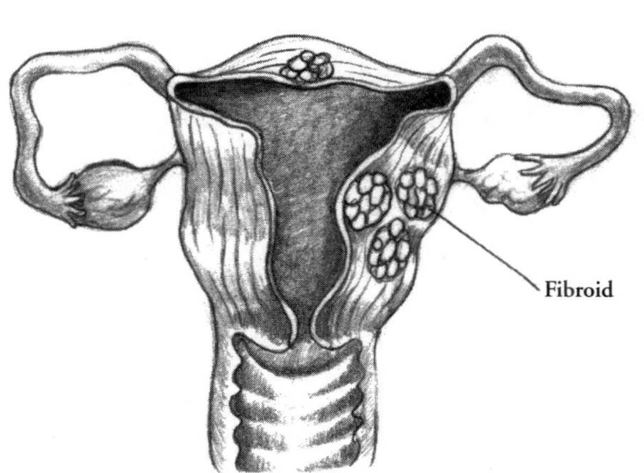

136

Q Are herbal remedies from the health food store successful for uterine fibroids?

A There is a prescription medication that usually shrinks fibroids, but they grow back to their initial size within three months of stopping the medication. Surgery or menopause are the only cures for symptomatic fibroids. At this time, there are no herbs known to be effective in treating fibroids.

137

Q Is there anything a woman can do if she finds it painful to have sex after a hysterectomy?

A A woman should be able to have normal intercourse without pain after a hysterectomy. However, the vagina may be tender and dry due to lack of hormones if the ovaries were removed and estrogen replacement therapy was not started. Complications of surgery can cause the vagina to be shorter. Vaginal dilators, estrogen replacement, the use of a lubricant, and a different position during intercourse may be helpful. Consult your physician if any of the problems persist.

138

Q Do birth control pills help older women with irregular periods?

A Healthy, low-risk, nonsmoking women can take lowdose oral contraceptives until menopause. Taking these medications during perimenopause has several potential advantages such as regular, light, predictable menses. These women can essentially "skip" the perimenopause symptoms of cycle irregularity and heavy bleeding. Birth control pills suppress hot flushes, maximize bone strength, decrease the risk of ovarian and uterine cancer, provide excellent contraception, and decrease menstrual cramps. Two low-dose pills are Alesse (Wyeth/Ayerst) and LoEstrin 1/20 (Parke-Davis). Not everyone can take oral contraceptives during perimenopause. Discuss this alternative with your health-care provider.

139

Q Why would a women develop uterine polyps late in life?

A Although there is no known cause for polyps (benign fingerlike growths), growth may be encouraged by irritation such as a chronic infection or chronic inflammation.

140

Q How are polyps treated?

A Polyps are usually treated by removing them from the mouth of the uterus by twisting them off at the base or from the uterine lining using a hysteroscope to cut the base of the polyp. Additional therapy is rarely needed.

141

Q What is a hysteroscopy?

A The hysteroscope is a fiber-optic lens system used to look inside the uterus for diagnostic testing. The instrument has openings to place instruments through to allow surgery while viewing. The cervix is dilated to allow the passage of this instrument. No incisions are necessary. Using a video camera to project the image of the uterine cavity on a television screen, the surgeon can detect any abnormal growths or tumors. Polyps, fibroids, scars, or any tissue suspicious for malignant or premalignant changes can be removed.

142

Q What's the difference between a total and partial hysterectomy?

A A total hysterectomy refers to the surgery that removes the body and mouth (cervix) of the uterus. Years ago some surgeons used to remove the body of the uterus and leave the mouth in place. This is called a partial, or subtotal, hysterectomy. Women with this type of surgery continue to be at risk for cervical cancer. Recently, there has been some renewed interest in the partial hysterectomy. A study in Sweden showed that sexual response might be better in women who still had their cervix while other studies did not support the finding. Most women who have a total hysterectomy are pleased with their sexual response after surgery if they have adequate estrogen replacement.

143

Q Why are some women so miserable after their hysterectomies?

A A hysterectomy is major surgery, and it should not be done if a more conservative treatment would be successful. However, with modern anesthesia and surgical techniques, hysterectomies are safer than ever. The majority of women who have hysterectomies experience no complications and are pleased with the results.

There are some women who have a strong psychological attachment to their uterus, feeling that the menstrual cycle and the ability to have children are an integral part of being female. These women may experience a sense of loss or the feeling that they are somehow incomplete after their uterus is removed. These feelings are intensified if the woman has not resolved her desire for future children. For women who experience these feelings, it is advisable to begin counseling before surgery. Remember also that the term "hysterectomy" applies only to the removal of the uterus. If the ovaries are also removed, a woman may experience estrogen withdrawal symptoms unless she takes estrogen replacement therapy.

144

Q How can a woman decide if a hysterectomy is right for her?

A Review the treatments you've had with your doctor and ask about other options. Have all alternative therapies been tried? Seek a second opinion from a qualified physician. If cancer or certain types of premalignant changes are present, a hysterectomy may be the only safe choice. Assess the impact of your gynecological problem on your quality of life. Because this is a big decision, don't hesitate to discuss any concerns, including sexual changes and surgical risks, with your physician. Most women who decide to have a hysterectomy are pleased with the final result.

145

Q Should a woman be concerned about some spotting after intercourse?

A Spotting after intercourse is sometimes due to a minor cervical infection, a vaginal infection, or a polyp. Some serious problems such as cervical cancer can cause spotting. It is best to see your health-care provider if you have spotting on a regular basis to be certain there is nothing serious causing the bleeding.

6

Osteoporosis

146

Q What is osteoporosis?

A Osteoporosis is bone thinning that results in structural failure of the skeleton and increased risk of bone fracture. It is a preventable disease. It is estimated that there are seventeen million women in the United States with untreated osteoporosis. Four out of ten women over age fifty will have a fracture due to osteoporosis during their remaining lifetime. This is a silent disease until a fracture occurs. As the Baby Boomers age, the number of women with osteoporosis increases each year.

147

Q Do men get osteoporosis?

A The main cause of osteoporosis is the loss of estrogen at the time of menopause. Estrogen is extremely important in keeping bones strong and healthy. Although men have a gradual decline in testosterone as they age, they don't go through a sudden loss of their sex hormones the way women do. Men who develop osteoporosis usually aren't diagnosed until after age seventy, and it usually isn't as severe.

148

Q At what age do women tend to get osteoporosis?

A Bone is lost quickly at menopause if estrogen replacement isn't used. The older and further away from menopause a woman is, the higher her risk of osteoporosis. As women reach their seventies, they usually experience the results of the disease. Certain medications, especially steroids or too much thyroid, can cause osteoporosis. People with rheumatoid arthritis are especially at risk and need to be carefully followed for bone thinning at an early age.

149

Q Are there symptoms to osteoporosis?

A Osteoporosis is a silent disease without symptoms until fractures start to occur. Once they begin to occur in the spine, pain may be a prominent symptom. The key to this disease is prevention and early detection.

150

Q Why do some women seem to shrink as they age?

A People with osteoporosis get shorter once the spinal fractures start to occur. Collapse of the supporting structure of the spine causes the decrease in height. This is not reversible, but there are therapies that will strengthen the bones and stop additional fractures and further loss of height.

151

Q What are the risk factors for osteoporosis?

A Asian and Caucasian women have a higher risk for osteoporosis than other ethnic groups. Other risk factors include the use of certain medications such as excessive thyroid, prednisone, or other steroids; family history of osteoporosis; menopause without estrogen replacement; early or premature menopause; low calcium intake; thin or small frame, low body weight; sedentary lifestyle; tobacco use; and excessive alcohol consumption.

152

Q Who should have a bone density test?

A Ideally, every woman should have a bone density test at or about fifty years old. This baseline test can determine the risk of future osteoporosis. If necessary, therapy can be started to prevent or stop the loss of bone. Women who are at high risk should definitely be screened, and others should discuss the testing with their physician.

153

Q How is a bone density test performed?

A The DEXA bone density test is completely painless and is one of the easiest medical tests you will ever have. You should wear comfortable clothes that don't have any metal buckles or buttons. Food can be eaten on the day of the test, but don't take a calcium supplement that day. The technician will ask you to lie quietly on a table, usually with your knees supported by a pillow. The DEXA uses about one-tenth the radiation exposure of a chest X ray as it determines the bone density of your hip and spine. The test will take about thirty to forty-five minutes, and the results are sent to your physician.

154

Q Are there different types of bone density tests?

A There are many types of bone density tests available and more are in development. Because of the increasing number of people at risk for osteoporosis, the industry is trying to find a less expensive and more convenient way to screen for bone loss. DEXA is the best test available. It can measure the density of the hip and the lumbar spine with reliable accuracy and little radiation exposure. If only one site is to be measured, the hip is the most important. Spinal fractures certainly cause problems, but it is usually the hip fracture that causes major disability and usually leads to nursing home admissions. The heel density is a good predictor of the density of the hip. Portable, less expensive machines that measure the density of the heel will be available soon.

155

Q At what age should a woman have a bone density test?

A Ideally, a bone density test is done when menopause begins, at about fifty years old. Bone is lost rapidly during the first five years after menopause. If menopause starts at an early age, a baseline bone density should be done at that time. A bone density should also be done if a bone fracture occurs without good reason.

156

Q What happens if a bone density test shows some problems?

A The bone density test will compare your bones to those of a thirty-five-year-old woman as well as other women your age. Ideally, bones would stay as strong as they were at thirty-five as we age. If there is bone thinning (osteopenia) that is significant but not bad enough to be called osteoporosis, you need to optimize your calcium, vitamin D, exercise, and consider starting estrogen replacement therapy. Discuss with your physician the option of taking a low dose of alendronate (Fosamax) to help prevent additional bone loss. If you have severe enough bone loss to be diagnosed with osteoporosis, you will need to take a more aggressive approach to prevent a fracture. In addition to the above measures, your doctor will probably recommend a full dose of Fosamax to help rebuild bone strength.

157

Q Is osteoporosis hereditary?

A A family history of osteoporosis definitely increases the risk of having the disease. However, osteoporosis is a preventable disorder. All women should be certain they have good calcium intake starting in childhood, stay active with an exercise program, and take vitamin D—400-800 IU daily. (Do not take more than this unless advised by your doctor; too much vitamin D is toxic.) A woman should strongly consider hormone replacement therapy when perimenopause transition begins and have her bone density measured about the time she starts menopause to provide a baseline. Also discuss with your physician the various drugs available to prevent and help reverse osteoporosis.

158

Q Are there medications that increase the risk of osteoporosis?

A There are many medications that can increase the risk of bone thinning. Probably the most common is thyroid supplementation for hypothyroidism. If you have low thyroid, you want to normalize your hormone levels. However, too much can lead to bone loss. It is important to monitor your TSH levels through a blood test prescribed by your physician. Prednisone or a similar steroid taken for rheumatoid arthritis, uncontrolled asthma, or certain connective tissue disorders can cause dramatic bone thinning. Women taking these medications should have their bone density checked early in life and may need preventative therapy for bone loss with Fosamax even before menopause occurs.

159

Q What type of exercise is best to increase bone strength?

A Any weight-bearing exercise, such as walking, will help maintain bone strength. People who are sedentary lose bone rapidly. Swimming is a good cardiovascular exercise but doesn't help bone strength. The best exercise for your bones is weight training either with free weights or with the machines used for circuit training. This type of exercise does have some risk of injury. If you already have osteoporosis, a physical therapist is probably the best professional to design and help you implement a weight-training program. Some stress improves bones, but too much stress hurts them. If you have normal bone density or only a mild decrease, a personal trainer should be able to help you organize a program and monitor your progress.

160

Q Why do some older women look so bent over that they have a hump on their back?

A The humped back appearance of some older women is called a dowager's hump and is the direct result of osteoporosis. The body bends forward as the spine collapses from fractures of the vertebrae. The bending stance squeezes the chest and abdomen causing breathing problems; she has difficulty inflating her lungs. During the course of normal aging, women lose a small amount of height. However, the major loss and dowager's hump are part of osteoporosis.

161

Q Why are there major complications after a simple hip fracture?

A Most women with hip fractures are over seventy years of age. A hip replacement is major surgery and some women have complications including blood clots, infection, and pneumonia. Almost 20 percent of the women with hip fractures die within one year due to the complications of surgery and prolonged bedrest. The older the person is, the more difficult the rehabilitation from hip surgery. Of the 80 percent who survive their fractures, nearly half require long-term nursing care for their disability. Whether the hip fractures first or a fall causes the fracture, women who stay in good physical condition are less likely to experience medical complications.

162

Q When should women start taking calcium supplements?

A Females need to began monitoring the calcium in their diet starting from adolescence and continuing through postmenopause. Most women are calcium deficient and need to use a supplement if they are not getting three calcium-rich food servings per day. The average woman needs 1,000 mg of calcium and usually gets about 600 mg from her diet.

163

Q What type of calcium is the best to take?

A Calcium citrate (Citracal) is an excellent type of calcium that can be taken on an empty stomach in the morning and doesn't require stomach acid for absorption. This is the best type of calcium if you take any medications to suppress stomach acid production. Calcium carbonate, such as the calcium in Tums, is another good form of calcium. It is chewable and should be taken with food.

164

Q Do you recommend that women take vitamin D supplements?

A It's recommended that women take 400-800 IU of vitamin D daily, because it assists with calcium absorption. However, the vitamin is toxic in high doses so any more than 800 IUs should not be taken unless prescribed by a doctor.

165

Q What is the treatment for osteoporosis?

A Once diagnosed through a bone density test, the woman and her medical-care provider will discuss options that include an exercise program, dietary changes, hormone replacement, and medications to stop the bone thinning process.

There are therapies to stop the progression of osteoporosis and several new medications to actually reverse osteoporosis. Estrogen supplementation is the main medical therapy to prevent additional bone loss. It is strongly recommended that a woman take estrogen replacement if she is able to.

Alendronate (Fosamax) has been approved for both the treatment and prevention of osteoporosis. Well-designed, double-blinded studies have shown not only progressive increases in bone density on DEXA scans but also an actual reduction in fractures. For at least four years after starting 10 mg of Fosamax daily, there have been continued increases in bone density. This medication must be taken exactly as directed for absorption. The patient has to take it with a full glass of plain water—no other fluid. She must not eat or take other medications, vitamins, or food for thirty minutes, and cannot lie down. The main complication of this medication is esophageal irritation due to reflux.

An alternate medication is calcitonin (Miacalcin). This hormone is naturally produced in the cells of the thyroid gland and encourages the incorporation of calcium into bone. Miacalcin is salmon calcitonin in a nasal spray. It is given as one puff in one nostril once daily. This drug is often helpful in relieving the pain of spinal fractures from osteoporosis. There is no fracture prevention data on calcitonin available to date.

A new form of slow-release fluoride will soon be available for the treatment of osteoporosis. The clinical studies suggest that it will be helpful in the treatment of the disease.

166

Q What's the relationship of estrogen and osteoporosis?

A Because estrogen is the major factor in preventing osteoporosis, there is rapid bone loss in some women within the first five years after menopause.

167

Q Why does osteoporosis cause pain?

A Osteoporosis pain is from spontaneous vertebra fractures. The spine actually starts to collapse, causing a decrease in height, the formation of a dowager's hump, and pain. The use of over-the-counter anti-inflammatory medications can help the pain if the woman can tolerate them. These preparations should be taken with food and a full glass of fluid. Salmon calcitonin (Miacalcin), which is an anti-osteoporosis drug, often provides relief. Since osteoporosis is a long-term, chronic condition, the use of narcotic pain killers is discouraged because of their addictive potential.

Aging Gracefully

168

Q Is plastic surgery a realistic option for any woman who wants to look younger?

A All surgery has risks, and plastic surgery is not a fountain of youth. But it is an option for most women who want to look as young as they feel. Before you make the decision to have plastic surgery, be realistic about what it can truly provide: It may be a quick makeover, but it will not have the long-term benefits of overall lifestyle changes. Healthy eating and an exercise or movement program will make you feel good on the inside and reflect in your mirror. The most detrimental thing you can do to your appearance (not to mention the harm to your health) is smoke or use tobacco in any way. It ruins your skin, adding about ten years to your appearance. Smoking can also rule out the possibility of a face-lift. Many plastic surgeons will not perform a face-lift on a smoker because the blood vessels in the skin are altered by smoking, increasing the risk of complications.

169

Q How old should a woman be before she considers having a face-lift?

A The condition of a woman's skin and her general health is more important than chronological age. Most cosmetic surgeons recommend a woman wait until at least age forty before considering the procedure.

170

Q How is a face-lift performed?

A Under local or general anesthesia, the surgeon makes an incision at the temple and continues to the front of the ear. The skin is then dissected free from the subcutaneous tissue and pulled back toward the ear. Excess skin is removed and the skin resutured. In some cases, the surgeon may tighten the facial muscles or remove excess fat. There is major swelling and bruising for two to three weeks after surgery. It often takes three to six months to see a complete healing and an optimal effect from the surgery. The average face-lift lasts six to eight years.

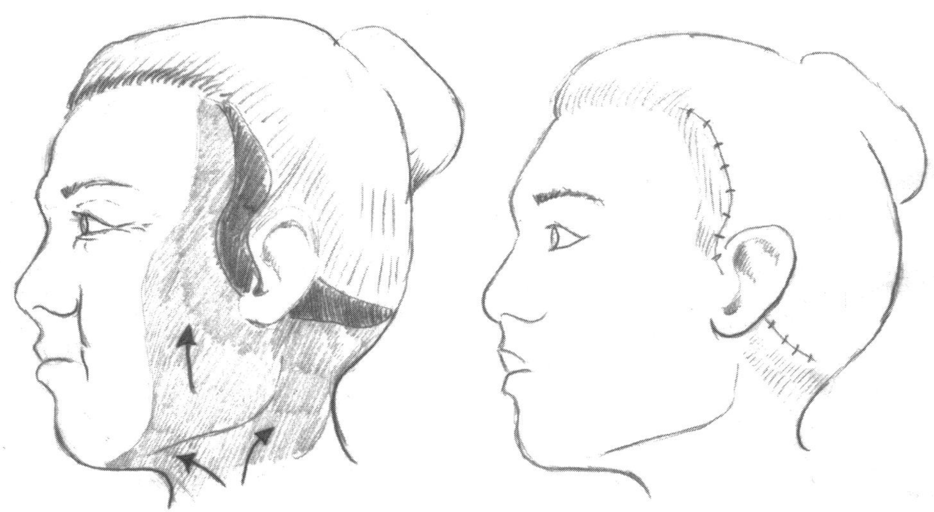

171

Q Why do some older women begin gaining a lot of weight even though they still eat the same way?

A As women age their metabolism starts to slow down. Unless there is an increase in exercise, most women over fifty will gain three to five pounds a year. Weight training adds muscle, which increases metabolism. Restricting food actually decreases the rate of metabolism. So developing a more consistent exercise program is a better way to fight weight gain than decreasing your calorie intake.

172

Q Does a woman's hair thin as she ages?

A There is a gradual overall hair thinning that comes with age. The amount of pubic and axillary hair can also decrease. Hair loss is not cause for concern, however, unless it is substantial. The most common reason for significant rapid hair loss in women is a low thyroid. If you are diagnosed with hypothyroidism and begin treatment with medication, your hair will return to its normal fullness in three to six months. If hypothyroidism is not the problem but you are still concerned that your hair loss is excessive, there are dermatologists who specialize in this. One option your dermatologist might recommend is Rogaine, which has been approved for treating hair loss in women. Rogaine must be prescribed by a physician and does not work for all hair loss.

173

Q How is laser resurfacing different from a chemical peel to help decrease facial lines?

A Laser resurfacing is one of the newest ways to remove scars and fine lines from the skin. The procedure needs to be done by a plastic surgeon, dermatologist, or physician with special training. A laser is used to remove the outer layers of the skin and smooth out defects in the skin surface.

A chemical peel is an excellent choice to erase acne scars from the skin. There are two kinds of chemical peels: superficial and deep. Basically, the procedure is to apply a chemical to the skin that causes the outer layer to come loose and slough off. The stronger the chemical and the longer it is applied, the deeper the peel. Although the results can be impressive, as with most surgeries and medical procedures, there is a risk of permanent damage. A chemical peel should only be performed by a specialist in plastic surgery or dermatology.

174

Q What is the best way to avoid aging skin?

A Sun is the number one cause of skin aging, followed by cigarette smoking. Avoid sun damage to the skin by using sunscreens, limiting direct sun exposure, and wearing protective clothing. And remember, tanning salons are probably not safer than basking in the direct sun.

175

Q Can the wrinkles be taken out of just the forehead?

A In order to remove the wrinkles from the forehead, the surgeon has to make an incision inside the hairline from one ear to the other. The skin is then dissected free from the subcutaneous tissue and the excess skin is trimmed away. The skin is then resutured in place. Some patients notice a difference in their hairline after this type of surgery.

176

Q What are the possible complications of a face-lift or brow-lift?

A A variety of complications can occur, such as excessive scarring, bleeding, formation of blood clots, infection from the surgical incisions, and damage to the facial nerve. Any woman who tends to form keloid scars, thick scars that result from the overgrowth of scar tissue, is not a good candidate for a face-lift, nor is a woman who smokes or has diabetes.

177

Q Can anything be done for droopy eyelids?

A Surgery to remove excess tissue and correct puffy eyes is called blepharoplasty. Sometimes this surgery is more than cosmetic since some women's eyelids droop so much that their vision is affected. A small horizontal incision is usually made in a crease of the upper or lower lids to hide the scar and excess tissue is removed. The fat pads under the eyes can be decreased to make the under eye less puffy. The woman is usually bruised and swollen for two to three weeks after this procedure.

178

Q What are the risks of liposuction?

A There have been some serious complications from the liposuction procedure. People with certain chronic illnesses are not good candidates. If an infection occurs in the area of the surgery, it can sometimes spread rapidly, causing sepsis, a life-threatening infection in the bloodstream, and even death. There can also be significant blood loss from this procedure. Scarring can occur, producing a "bumpy" surface.

Beware of doctors that try to oversell their services or the outcome. A board certified plastic surgeon with a good reputation in the community should be qualified to do the procedure.

179

Q What is the best way to select a surgeon to do a face-lift?

A Choosing the right plastic surgeon is the key to having a good experience. Make an appointment for a preliminary consultation with several physicians that have been referred by other doctors or friends. All of them should be board certified with The American Board of Plastic Surgery. Evaluate the hospitals they have privileges at and ask all of the questions you have regardless of how you think they may sound. Discuss the pros and cons of the procedure so you can make an informed decision.

180

Q What should older women do to make sure they keep their teeth?

A The dentist is the person we need to help us protect our teeth. Regular dental visits every six months will allow a woman to take care of problems when they arise. Gum disease is the most common reason to lose teeth, so taking good care of your gums is extremely important. Simply flossing daily is a key to good oral hygiene and gum health. Some mouth and tongue cancers can be detected by a dentist before symptoms may arise.

181

Q Why do some women develop unsightly veins in their legs as they age?

A Spider veins tend to occur in families. They are more obvious on pale skin, become more pronounced with age, and are aggravated by long hours of standing. Spider veins can be treated with sclerotherapy. It is a slow process that requires multiple treatments to be successful. The procedure calls for injecting a solution into the veins, which causes the walls to collapse. The amount of pain depends on the type of fluid that is inserted and the skill of the physician. Laser therapy is also helpful for removing small veins that can't be injected easily. It's important to find a physician who specializes in this procedure.

182

Q What can be done for the dark purple varicose veins?

A Varicose veins are often painful and should be treated. Injection solutions often aren't successful with larger varicose veins. In these cases, the vein has to be tied off and perhaps even stripped or removed. A general surgeon specializing in vascular surgery or a plastic surgeon are your best choices to perform this procedure.

183

Q How often should a woman have her skin checked for cancer?

A Fair-skinned people with extended sun exposure are at increased risk for skin cancer. Women with red hair are at special risk. Everyone should check her own skin monthly and have a dermatologist or family physician check it yearly. Any growth, mole, or lesion should be examined by a physician immediately if it bleeds or changes size or color.

184

Q How many hours of sleep does a woman need to function properly?

A The need for sleep varies from person to person. Some people function at top speed at five hours while others need nine. Many people try to fit two days worth of activities into one and find themselves sleep deprived. Signs of sleep deprivation include an inability to concentrate, irritability, anxiety, and depression. Adding as little as one hour a night might significantly increase your efficiency and tolerance of daily stresses.

Part III
A Look at the Body

The Female Breast

185

Q What is a breast?

A The breast is composed of glands, ducts, and fat. The glandular tissue is designed to produce milk, and ducts carry the milk to the nipple. As a woman ages, the breast tissues change form naturally. Breasts tend to have the same amount of glandular tissue no matter what their size. The difference in breast size is due to the fat between the gland units.

186

Q How important is it for a woman in her twenties to do a monthly breast self-exam?

A Ideally, you should start doing breast self-exams (BSE) when you start your menstrual cycles. Therefore, no woman is ever too young to start. Performing an exam on a regular monthly basis will enable you to notice any changes that might occur from month to month. It's important to know your own body.

187

Q When should the monthly breast exam be done?

A The ideal time to do an exam is three or four days after the end of your period if you are in the childbearing years because that's when there is the least amount of tenderness and swelling due to hormonal changes. Women who no longer menstruate should pick a day that's easy to remember and mark it on the calendar. The first day of the month is an easy one to remember.

188

Q What is the correct way to perform a breast self-exam?

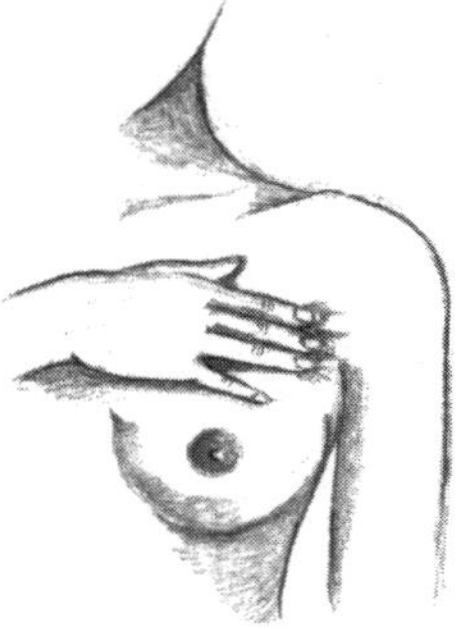

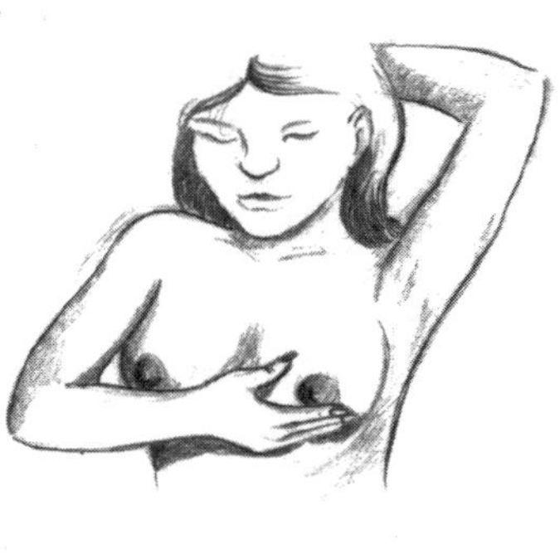

A The basic BSE method instructs a woman to use the fat pads of the three middle fingers to examine each breast in a circular pattern. Start near the collarbone and with small, circular motions move in toward the nipple. Check down to the bra line and from the armpit to the breastbone with both light and deep pressure. In the shower, soap each breast. Then with one arm raised, check the left breast and underarm area with the right hand and vice versa. Feel for any changes. An alternate method is to start with the nipple and check the breast in widening circles. Look for visual changes in the mirror with your arms at your sides, with your arms over your head, and with your hands clasped under your chin while flexing the chest muscles and bending forward with breasts hanging. Then, place a folded towel under the mid back while lying down. Repeat the fingertip exam of each breast in the circular pattern. Consult a health-care provider if you have any questions or suspect any changes.

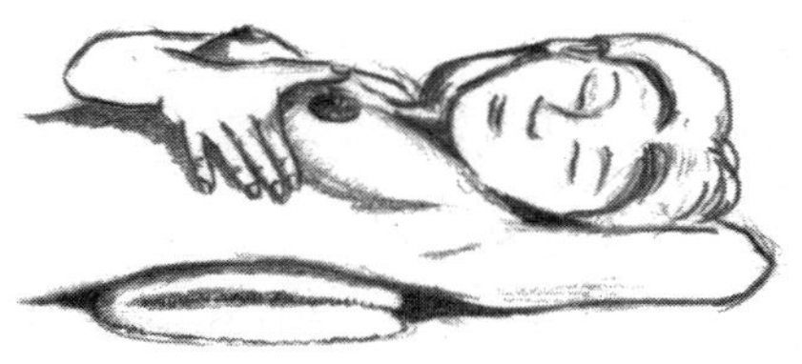

189

Q What is a mammogram?

A A mammogram is a special type of breast X ray designed to detect breast abnormalities before they can be felt. The radiation dose is small, allowing mammography to be used as a safe screening procedure.

190

Q Does a mammogram really hurt?

A In order to get good X rays, the breasts are compressed between two clear plastic shelves. Most women find this test slightly uncomfortable but not painful. Some women experience breast tenderness the week before their period, which could make the mammogram more uncomfortable. For that reason, it is better to schedule a mammogram after your period. If you are concerned about discomfort, take some acetaminophen before the procedure.

191

Q How accurate are mammograms?

A Although this is the best screening procedure available, it is not perfect in detecting all abnormalities. Most radiologists report a 94 percent efficiency for detection of a breast cancer.

192

Q Who should have a mammogram?

A Any woman who has a suspicious breast mass should have a mammogram. A woman should have a baseline mammogram between the ages of thirty-five and forty. She should then have one every one to two years from ages forty to fifty and every year after fifty, depending on risk factors.

193

Q Does a woman who has no history of cancer in her family still need to have a mammogram?

A Most women who develop breast cancer have no family history of the disease. All women with breasts should be screened on a regular basis.

194

Q What does "dense breasts" mean on a mammogram report?

A Dense breasts simply have more glandular tissue. Young women tend to have more glands compared to the aging woman. The denser the breast, the more difficult it is to read the mammogram and the easier it is for a lump, or abnormality, to hide undetected on the X ray. Dense breasts are not abnormal.

195

Q What is fibrocystic breast disease?

A Fibrocystic breasts are not actually diseased. They are often lumpy from swelling of the glands and tender to the touch. They may be worse just before a menstrual period.

Fibrocystic changes do not necessarily increase the risk of breast cancer. They can, however, make an abnormality harder to detect because of the natural lumpiness.

196

Q What is a breast ultrasound?

A A breast ultrasound, which has essentially no risk because there isn't any radiation, is not done on a routine basis. It is performed to determine if a mass is cystic or solid. Cysts are rarely malignant. Solid lesions have a higher risk. Ultrasound is sometimes used to examine lumps that can be felt but not seen on a mammogram.

197

Q Why are breast cysts aspirated?

A Some breast cysts are painful, and aspirating them relieves that pain. Breast cysts are aspirated in the office using a local anesthetic to numb the skin. Because cysts are filled with fluid, the doctor can use a needle and syringe to drain it. The doctor may send the fluid to a pathologist for study, but some doctors do not do this if the fluid is clear and doesn't contain any blood. After the fluid is removed, many cysts will not return.

198

Q If a woman is experiencing pain in her breasts, should she be concerned?

A Most breast pain is related to hormone changes in the body. Even though only 6 percent of patients with early breast cancer have pain, it is a good idea to see your physician for an evaluation.

199

Q Are there any options for relieving breast pain?

A There are medications such as Danazol and Tamoxifen which decrease breast tenderness but cause side effects. Many women find that taking evening primrose oil as a daily supplement significantly decreases the pain. It takes about three months to experience the full effect of primrose oil. You can take up to two 500 mg capsules twice daily. Evening primrose oil is available at most health food stores.

200

Q Is a breast lump always cancer?

A Actually, eight out of ten breast lumps are benign. But this is no reason to put off seeing your doctor if you find a lump in your breast. Early diagnosis of a breast cancer is the key to improved chances of a cure. You should always see your physician immediately for an evaluation if you have a persistent breast lump.

201

Q How long do doctors normally wait before doing a breast lump biopsy?

A Most clinicians feel it is safe to wait several menstrual cycles before performing a biopsy on a benign-feeling mass in a woman under thirty. In an older patient, especially if the mass feels suspicious or shows signs of cancer on the mammogram, a biopsy will be done immediately. Any enlarging or persistent mass should be biopsied whether it is seen on a mammogram or not.

202

Q Is breast cancer becoming more common?

A There has been a continual increase in the number of patients diagnosed with breast cancer since the early 1940s. Because age is a major risk factor for developing breast cancer and women are living longer today, the aging of the female population accounts for some of the increase. There is also the possibility that the increasing environmental toxins are playing a role in the increase in breast cancer, but this remains to be accurately studied and proven. Since 1980 we have seen an even steeper increase in diagnosing the disease as a direct result of improved early detection techniques. At the same time, we are finally beginning to see a decrease in the number of deaths caused by breast cancer.

203

Q What factors increase a woman's risk of developing breast cancer?

A Age is the greatest risk factor for breast cancer. Other risk factors include women who have a first-degree relative (such as a mother or sister or even a male relative) with the disease, breast cancer survivors who still have breast tissue, women who start menstrual cycles early and go through menopause late, and women who live in the United States or Europe. There is also some evidence that shows both giving birth and breastfeeding may slightly reduce the risk of breast cancer.

204

Q Do birth control pills increase the risk of getting breast cancer?

A There is no medical evidence that using birth control pills either increases or decreases the risk of breast cancer.

205

Q Does the size of a woman's breasts affect her chances of getting breast disease?

A Most breasts have about the same number of glands regardless of their size. Women with large breasts do not have a higher risk of disease. Large breasts, however, may make a diagnosis of a breast mass more difficult. Mammography, which X-rays breast tissue, may be even more important for early diagnosis in women with large breasts.

206

Q Why are we supposed to examine under our arms during a breast self-exam?

A Breast tissue goes all the way into the armpit (axilla). It is important to check this area, called the Tail of Spence, when you do a breast self-examination. Both benign and malignant breast tumors can develop here.

207

Q What is a breast biopsy?

A A breast biopsy is surgical removal of a small piece of suspicious breast tissue. It is sent to a pathologist to see if it contains cancer. The biopsy procedure is usually done as an outpatient or as a day surgery procedure. Usually either local anesthesia with sedation or a general anesthesia is used.

208

Q What's the difference between a biopsy and a lumpectomy?

A These procedures may be the same for small lesions. A biopsy implies that only part of the lesion, or lump, is removed for evaluation. A lumpectomy indicates that the entire lump, as well as the tissue surrounding it, is removed. For certain tumors, alumpectomy has been shown to be as effective as a simple mastectomy (removal of the breast).

209

Q What does negative lymph nodes mean?

A At the time of the initial surgery to remove a breast tumor, whether it is a lumpectomy or mastectomy, some of the lymph nodes in the armpit may be removed for evaluation. The lymph nodes are reported negative if no tumor tissue was detected. Negative lymph nodes suggest that the cancer has not spread from the breast to the rest of the body. It suggests a good prognosis.

210

Q Is a woman cured of cancer if she had a lumpectomy five years ago?

A The longer the distance a survivor is from the cancer diagnosis, the greater the chance of permanent remission. However, physicians now consider eight years disease free as a cure.

211

Q What's the difference between a radical, a modified, and a simple mastectomy?

A A radical mastectomy was performed before anyone knew how breast cancer spreads. In this scenario, the entire breast, chest wall muscles, fat, and lymph node tissues were removed all the way into the armpit. This was a disfiguring surgery that left a scar to cover the chest wall bones. A modified radical approach is when the surgeon removes the breast and all of the fatty tissue and lymph nodes. A simple mastectomy is when the breast and a sampling of lymph nodes are taken. In addition to checking for cancer cells, the lymph node removal tends to decrease the flow of lymph from the arm, which often results in swelling of the arm.

212

Q Why would one person be getting chemotherapy for breast cancer when another isn't?

A The therapy for breast cancer is individualized for each woman. Treatment options are dependent on the woman's preference, the size of the tumor, the health and age of the woman, and whether or not the cancer has spread to other sites. If there is no cancer detected outside the breast, chemotherapy usually isn't indicated.

213

Q Should reconstruction be done at the same time as a mastectomy?

A Many women choose to have reconstruction at the same time as they have their mastectomy. The new breast tissue can be formed from natural tissue taken from the back or abdomen. In some cases, a saline implant is used. The more natural tissue that can be used, the more natural the result. Others prefer to go through breast cancer therapy, including radiation and chemotherapy if needed, and delay reconstruction of their breast. Some women decide not to have reconstruction in order to avoid additional surgery. A breast prosthesis can give a natural-looking result through clothing.

214

Q What's the difference between silicone and saline breast implants?

A Silicone implants are hollow shells filled with silicone gel-like material. Saline implants are filled with sterile salt water. Most people feel that silicone implants have a more natural feel, but there is a risk that the shell will rupture, allowing the silicone gel to seep out into the tissue. A saline implant can also rupture, but it releases only harmless salt water. Ruptures are uncommon, but if one does occur, the old implant must be removed and can be replaced by a new one. The saline implant shells are made of silicone, but they are not a danger because it is the fluid that is released from within the shell during a rupture that seeps into the tissue.

215

Q Do breast implants cause diseases?

A There is no medical evidence that breast implants cause any type of cancer. However, silicone implants that rupture allow silicone to seep out into the tissues. This can cause scarring and pain. There has been a great deal of debate about whether silicone can cause immune system disorders.

216

Q How likely are you to get cancer in another female organ if you've had breast cancer?

A There are families in which breast and ovarian cancer are both prevalent. Medical science has recently identified a gene that indicates the risk of someone getting both breast and ovarian cancer. Until more information is known, most physicians evaluate the family history to determine probable risk for these cancers.

217

Q Is there a relationship between bone density and breast cancer?

A Recent studies have suggested that women with good bone density may have an increased risk of breast cancer. It may be that the exposure to estrogen, which increases the strength of the bones, increases the risk of breast cancer. More studies are needed to determine whether this association is true.

218

Q What can a breast cancer survivor do about dryness during intercourse if she's not taking estrogen?

A Using a lubricant helps some women with vaginal dryness during intercourse. Solid vegetable Crisco is one option. There are several products developed just as sexual lubricants including Astroglide, Replens, Vagisil Intimate Moisturizer, and K-Y Jelly. Estring provides a small amount of local estrogen to the vaginal tissues without significantly increasing long-term blood levels. It is inserted into the vagina and gradually releases small amounts of estrogen. This product is not approved for breast cancer patients, but some clinicians are suggesting that it may be the safest estrogen alternative available. Eli Lilly has trials going on in twenty-five countries for raloxifene, an alternative to traditional hormone therapy. A local antibiotic cream may help decrease tenderness if there is a chronic infection. Contact your physician if dryness continues.

219

Q What is Tamoxifen?

A Tamoxifen is a well-tolerated drug that may decrease the risk of future breast cancer by blocking estrogen receptors in the breast. Some women experience hot flushes while taking this medication. If a woman with a uterus takes the drug, she has a slight increase in risk for developing uterine (endometrial) cancer. A physician should monitor a woman taking Tamoxifen for irregular vaginal bleeding. Trials in the U.S. and England also show the medication to have some benefit in the prevention of osteoporosis.

220

Q Can a woman have a healthy baby after undergoing chemotherapy?

A Chemotherapy agents can destroy the eggs in the ovaries. It may take the ovaries many months or years to recover from the toxic effects of the drugs. Some women never recover ovarian function after chemotherapy. Only time will let the woman know if future fertility is possible.

221

Q Can a woman who's had breast cancer take estrogen safely?

A Although estrogen is important in the prevention of heart disease and osteoporosis, there is a great deal of controversy over its use by breast cancer survivors. Each woman, in partnership with her physician, must assess the potential risks of the drug compared to the benefits.

222

Q Why would a woman be leaking fluid from her breasts if she wasn't pregnant or breastfeeding?

A Unexpected production of fluid from the breast needs to be investigated by a physician. This inappropriate production of fluid is most often due to an imbalance of the hormone prolactin or a decreased production of thyroid hormone. Some tumors of the breast can also cause fluid discharge.

223

Q Can any woman breastfeed her baby?

A It is rare for a woman not to be able to breastfeed her baby. Most women can provide total nutrition for their babies for the first three months of life or more. However, breastfeeding doesn't allow the easy monitoring of a bottle to determine whether the baby is getting an adequate supply of nourishment. Your doctor, pediatrician, or a lactation specialist can teach you how to monitor how much milk your baby is getting. Breastfeeding is a system that has worked for millions of years.

224

Q Is it harmful to a baby not to breastfeed?

A Although everyone agrees breastfeeding is a good way to feed your baby and pass on some immunities, it isn't the only way. Infants who are bottlefed with plenty of love and nurturing do just as well as breastfed babies. Women who choose not to breastfeed can feel confident their babies will be healthy and well nourished by formula bottlefeeding.

225

Q What are the advantages of breastfeeding?

A Human milk is optimum for babies, because of the natural immunities it provides. Antibodies from the mother are transferred to her baby. It also helps the mother by encouraging the uterus to return to its normal size. There is also the advantage of not having to prepare formula and clean bottles.

226

Q Are there certain women who shouldn't breastfeed?

A There are few contraindications to breastfeeding. Women who are ill or are taking medication, which could harm the baby, should not breastfeed. If you are concerned about whether or not it's okay for you to breastfeed, ask you doctor.

227

Q Does breastfeeding come naturally or does a woman need to be taught how?

A Breastfeeding education should begin a month or two prior to delivery. There will be a nurse available in the hospital who is trained in breastfeeding education. A woman has to believe in the system and educate herself. It is helpful to talk with other women who have successfully breastfed their children. Discuss the process with friends and family or contact the La Leche League in your area.

228

Q How do you know when the baby is getting enough breast milk?

A The baby is getting enough milk if diapers are being changed four or more times a day and the baby isn't getting any supplemental fluids by bottle. In addition, normal weight gain will indicate the baby is getting plenty of food. The mother's milk supply is controlled by how much the baby sucks. If the baby is getting a supplemental bottle, he or she won't suck enough at the breast to keep the milk control system working.

229

Q What is mastitis?

A Mastitis is a breast infection that occurs most often during pregnancy or breastfeeding. The tissue of the breast may become infected with a staph bacteria. The breast will become tender, red, and swollen. The mother often has fever and needs to be treated with an antibiotic, warm compresses, and mild pain medication. Most of the time the problem can be resolved and you can continue to breastfeed.

The Reproductive Organs

230

Q Why would a woman always seem to have a vaginal discharge on her underwear?

A The vagina cleans itself constantly. The outer cells fall off as new cells form. Hormonal changes during the menstrual cycle also affect the cells of the vagina. Estrogen increases the division and growth of vaginal cells, which increases the production of a clear, egg white-like mucus from the cells inside the mouth of the uterus (endocervical cells). The amount and type of vaginal discharge can change during the cycle due to hormonal changes. The surge of estrogen prior to ovulation produces increased amounts of clear, stringy mucous, which is optimal for sperm transport. After egg release, under the influence of progesterone, the vaginal discharge becomes white and "tacky," like whipped egg whites. A normal discharge does not cause burning, pain, or itching. You should see your physician if you are experiencing any of these symptoms.

231

Q How does a woman know when to see the doctor and when it's okay to use an over-the-counter preparation?

A Over-the-counter products to treat vaginal symptoms have limited usefulness. The vaginal creams and suppositories that are advertised to treat odor and itching are only masking symptoms; they are not treating the cause. They should be used as a temporary source of relief of symptoms until you can see a health-care provider. Natural vaginal secretions should not have a foul odor. It is reasonable to use an over-the-counter preparation for a yeast infection if you have the typical symptoms of a cottage cheese-like discharge and itching. It's time to see a health-care provider if the symptoms are not cleared up after one cycle of over-the-counter treatments. Some yeast infections are resistant to over-the-counter therapies. See a physician if you have abdominal pain, pain with urination, or fever.

232

Q What can a woman do to protect her underwear from a discharge?

A A mini pad can be worn to protect underwear. Pads with deodorants can cause allergic reactions such as rashes and should be avoided.

233

Q What can a woman do about an embarrassing itch that's driving her crazy?

A There are a number of possible causes for itching around the opening to the vagina and the perianal area. A vaginal yeast infection is a common cause of itching. If one treatment

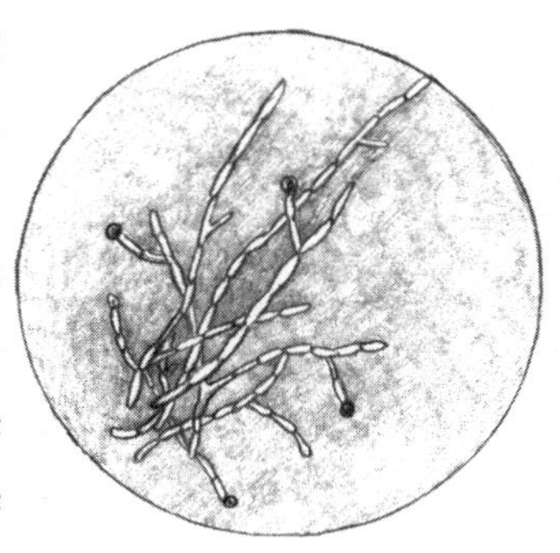

with an over-the-counter yeast product doesn't work, see your health-care provider for an examination and microscopic vaginal smear. Skin disorders, such as psoriasis, can affect this area of the body, too. If there are young children in the house, and the itching seems to be worse at night or early in the morning, the diagnosis could be pinworms. A doctor must prescribe medication and a course of action to clear this condition. Persistent itching of the skin of the vulva sometimes indicates a precancerous or cancerous change. A visit to your health-care provider will alleviate any concerns.

234

Q If a woman is treated for a vaginal infection, should her partner also be treated?

A The partners of women who have a trichomonas vaginal infection should definitely be treated. However, there is no indication that treating a partner when a woman has a yeast infection is helpful. Bacterial vaginitis can be sexually transmitted, but women who are not sexually active can also get this infection. Studies don't clearly indicate that treating partners in a bacterial vaginal infection is useful. The physician may suggest treatment for a partner if there is trouble clearing the infection or if it is recurring.

235

Q Does pelvic pain with a vaginal discharge indicate a problem?

A Pelvic pain can be a sign of a serious problem such as pelvic inflammatory disease, a urinary tract infection, appendicitis, or an ovarian cyst among others. If you are experiencing only vaginal symptoms without pelvic or abdominal pain, you can try one round of over-the-counter therapy. If the symptoms are not cured or the problem recurs within two months, see your doctor. If you are having more serious pelvic pain with vaginal discharge (or a burning sensation when you urinate), you should see a physician immediately.

236

Q How should a woman decide if she should douche?

A The vagina naturally cleans itself on a regular basis. Douching is not necessary and provides an opportunity to introduce agents into the body that might cause an allergic reaction. See a doctor if you are douching because of bad vaginal odor. Douching should never be done more than twice in one week.

237

Q What should a woman use for a douche?

A A mild vinegar and water solution should be used if a woman chooses to douche. The disposable, over-the-counter douches are safer to use because they are only used once and can't harbor germs for infection.

238

Q How should the outside lips of the vagina be cleaned?

A The outer lips of the vagina are called the labia. They should be cleaned with a mild, nondrying, nondeodorant soap and warm water. Cetaphil and Aveeno are good choices. Don't use antiseptic agents such as Betadine for routine cleansing because the tissue is delicate and sensitive to excessive drying. Limit the use of soap on the labia to once a day and use warm water if you want a second cleaning. See a medical provider if the skin in this area seems excessively dry or irritated or if there is a vaginal odor.

239

Q What are the most common causes of vaginal infections?

A The four common causes of vaginal infections are bacterial vaginosis (*gardenerella vaginalis* and other bacteria), yeast (*candida albicans* or other candida species), trichomonas (single-cell parasite), and atrophic vaginitis.

Bacterial vaginosis (BV) is the most common cause of vaginal infections in women of reproductive age. Although it can be asymptomatic, some women complain of an increased thin, white or gray vaginal discharge, vaginal irritation, and an unpleasant, fishy odor. Vaginal intercourse and menses can sometimes aggravate these symptoms. BV is commonly found in women who have more serious pelvic infections and can be sexually transmitted.

Although women think yeast infections are the most common type of vaginal infection, yeast is really only the cause of about one-third of these infections. The symptoms of a yeast infection are itching; redness, which can extend to the anal area and groin; a thick, white, cottage cheese-like discharge; and little or no odor. There are four conditions that increase the chance of a yeast infection: antibiotics, diabetes, pregnancy, and AIDS.

Trichomonas vaginitis is caused by the sexual transmission of a single-cell parasite. It is often asymptomatic in men. A woman may experience severe itching, intense redness of the vaginal tissues, and an unpleasant odor. The vaginal discharge may be profuse and is sometimes frothy and discolored. Intercourse and urination may both be painful. Both sexual partners should be treated for trichomonas, and it is recommended that you be screened for other sexually transmitted diseases.

Atrophic vaginitis, in which the vaginal tissues become thin and fragile, occurs if a woman doesn't have adequate levels of estrogen. Because of the lack of estrogen, the healthy acidity of the vagina is lost, suppressing the growth of healthy bacteria. An overgrowth of abnormal bacteria results, producing a foul odor. Other symptoms include decreased lubrication and a profuse, watery, yellow or gray discharge. The best treatment for atrophic vaginitis is local or systemic estrogen therapy.

240

Q What causes recurrent vaginal infections?

A It may appear that vaginal infections are recurring when in fact they were never cured but only suppressed. See a physician for a vaginal smear and perhaps culture to determine the specific cause of the infection. Once the cause is determined, the proper treatment can be prescribed.

241

Q What can a woman do for a discharge with an odor?

A Because there are so many different types of infections that may be the culprit, it is important to see a health-care provider who can do a complete pelvic examination, test the secretions for the cause, and prescribe the proper medication. Covering up the problem with a douche or using over-the-counter treatments only mask the symptoms, and you need to solve the problem.

242

Q What can be done to alleviate a dry and irritated vaginal area?

A A dry feeling in the vaginal area can be the result of inadequate estrogen levels, a vaginal infection, or a skin disorder. Don't use perfumed products; instead, cleanse the area with a mild, nondeodorant soap and warm water daily for relief. The vaginal area can be lubricated with a product like Replens. A sexual lubricant such as Astroglide or even plain Crisco solid shortening can be used during intercourse. Contact a physician if the dryness persists.

243

Q If a woman is experiencing painful intercourse, could her vagina be too small?

A It is rare for a vagina to be too small for comfortable sexual intercourse. If the woman has adequate foreplay to produce natural lubrication, the tissues will stretch without discomfort. A sexual lubricant can be used or vaginal dilators can be used at home to increase the size of the opening. Sometimes the vagina is decreased in size by a hysterectomy or repair of a weakness between the rectum and the vagina or the bladder and the vagina. A physician can work with a patient to alleviate the problem.

244

Q Is something wrong if intercourse is painful deep inside?

A Painful intercourse is called dysparunia. Persistent pain with deep penetration may be due to a pelvic infection, fibroids, pelvic adhesions, scarring, or endometriosis. Before seeing a physician for persistent pain, try a lubricant with intercourse and keep a diary of when the pain occurs. A diary will help determine if the problem is related to something like a certain sexual position, a certain time of the month, or inadequate foreplay. If the lubricant doesn't help, see your doctor. She may do a pelvic exam, cultures for sexually transmitted diseases, a Pap smear, and a pelvic ultrasound. She will probably begin with conservative therapies, but if they are not successful, a laparoscopy may be necessary.

245

Q Is it safe to use the sprays and powders you find in the personal products section at the pharmacy or grocery store?

A A gentle, nondrying soap and warm water is all that's needed to be clean and healthy. The use of talc on the genital area increases the risk of ovarian cancer. There is no medical value to such personal products. In fact, they may be masking an odor indicative of a medical problem.

246

Q What is the best lubricant to use during intercourse?

A The best vaginal lubricant is solid, white Crisco shortening. It has no perfume, preservatives, or coloring. It is a chemically pure vegetable product is inexpensive, and provides excellent lubrication. However, because the product is oil based, it may stain bedsheets and clothing. There are a variety of lubricants that can be purchased over the counter in a pharmacy or grocery store. Replens, a vaginal moisturizer that can be inserted into the vagina several times a week at bedtime, stays in the vagina for several days providing lubrication when needed. Astroglide is a good choice for a water-soluble lubricant that can be used at the time of intercourse.

247

Q Why is eating yogurt or taking acidophilus beneficial?

A Naturally cultured yogurt and acidophilus contain lactobacillus, a healthy bacteria that keeps the vaginal environment in balance. The healthy vagina has an acid pH that inhibits the growth of unhealthy bacteria and yeast and encourages the growth of lactobacillus. The pH of the vagina is extremely important for vaginal health. Eating naturally cultured yogurt or taking acidophilus may be helpful in keeping the microorganisms in the gastrointestinal track in balance.

248

Q What is the cervix?

A The cervix is the mouth of the uterus, which projects into the vagina. This structure, which feels like the tip of the nose, can be felt by inserting fingers into the vagina. It is the cervix that must dilate for a baby to pass from the uterus into the vagina during labor. The Pap smear is taken from around the opening of the cervix.

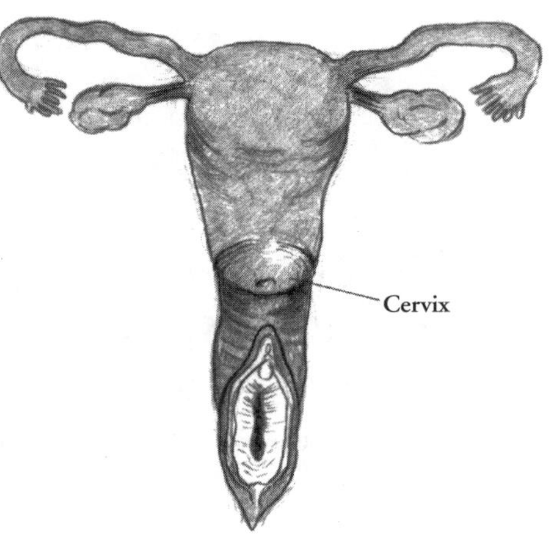

249

Q What is a Pap smear for?

A The Pap smear is a screening test to detect cervical cancer before a problem can be detected by a visual examination. Cervical cancer was the number-one killer of women in the Western world before the Pap smear. The disease can now be detected early and treated in a precancerous condition. The Pap smear is one of the success stories of modern medicine. Every woman with a uterus should have one yearly.

250

Q What causes an abnormal Pap smear?

A Mildly abnormal Pap smears can be caused by irritation from a minor vaginal infection or by an early stage of premalignant cell changes. Most, if not all, cases of precancerous and cancerous changes are from a papilloma virus. Women with papilloma virus are at increased risk for cervical cancer and should be closely monitored.

251

Q How could a woman whose Pap smear was normal be diagnosed with cervical cancer?

A A Pap smear is only a screening tool and is not 100 percent accurate. Even the best laboratories in the country have a 10 to 15 percent false negative rate. There are many new techniques, such as PapNet, that are becoming available to increase the accuracy of Pap smears.

252

Q Why would a doctor do a colposcopy after an abnormal Pap smear?

A A Pap smear is a screening tool and not a diagnostic test. The Pap is like a red flag that tells the physician that something is wrong and additional testing is necessary to determine the cause of the abnormal cells. The best test to evaluate the cause of an abnormal Pap smear is a colposcopy.

൦ 253 ൦

Q What is a colposcopy?

A A colposcope is an optical instrument that acts like a magnifying glass or a microscope on a stand. The patient is placed in the position used for a Pap smear, and a speculum is inserted into the vagina to allow the physician to see the cervix. A dilute vinegar solution is usually dabbed onto the cervix. It feels cool but doesn't cause any pain. By looking through the colposcope, which is on a stand, the physician can look carefully and examine the cervix for any abnormal areas. If she does see abnormal tissue, she may do a biopsy to remove a small piece of tissue to be studied by a pathologist. If a biopsy is done, it feels like a quick, sharp pinch. A colposcopy and biopsy, if necessary, allow the physician to determine the cause of an abnormal Pap smear and whether any additional treatment will be required.

൦ 254 ൦

Q Why would someone need a cone biopsy?

A Sometimes the physician is unable to see the area of the cervix that needs to be evaluated because it's far inside the canal or opening of the cervix. In this event, a cone-shaped piece of tissue is removed during a day surgery procedure and sent to the pathologist who studies it under the microscope. The pathologist will tell the surgeon how severe the problem is and whether or not all the abnormal tissue was removed.

255

Q What is a LEEP procedure?

A The loop electrical excision procedure is a new way to do a cone biopsy. A wire loop with an electrical current flowing through it is used to remove tissue in the cone shape instead of a surgeon using a scalpel or scissors.

256

Q Why would a doctor use a laser to treat abnormal cervical tissue?

A A laser can be used interchangeably with the other surgical tools. However, many surgeons find using the laser takes a long time. It has no advantages over the traditional scalpel or scissors and can't compete with the speed of the LEEP procedure.

257

Q What is cryosurgery?

A Cryosurgery is when the opening or canal of the cervix is frozen to remove abnormal tissue. Since cold is a natural anesthetic, the patient usually feels cramping while an ice ball forms in the area. The tissue is usually frozen and thawed twice. The freezing causes the outer cells to fall off and be replaced by healthy new cells that grow from the deeper tissues.

258

Q Can a woman still become pregnant and carry a baby after having treatment for an abnormal Pap smear?

A Most women who have had tissue removed from their cervix remain fertile and are able to have children. Sometimes the amount of cervical mucus for sperm transport into the uterus is decreased after one of these procedures. It's also possible for the cervix to be weakened by the removal of tissue. Both problems can be addressed by insemination of the partner's sperm or using surgery to strengthen the mouth of the uterus.

259

Q What is cervical dysplasia?

A Dysplasia is a precancerous change of the cervix that is graded, or rated, as mild, moderate, or severe. Sometimes the dysplasia can cure or reverse itself and become normal tissue again. The more severe the dysplasia, the less likely the change back to normal and the more likely it will progress to cancer.

260

Q What is cervical carcinoma in situ?

A Carcinoma in situ means that the cells appear cancerous but have not spread outside the superficial layer of the cervix. This cancer is curable by simply removing the abnormal tissue because the cells have not spread.

261

Q Is cervical cancer a preventable disease?

A Avoidance of the papilloma virus, which is believed to be the cause of the disease, is the best way to escape cervical cancer. Men can carry the papilloma virus and not be aware of it. Limiting sexual partners and using condoms until a monogamous relationship is achieved will help avoid the virus.

262

Q Why would it be necessary to have a hysterectomy because of cervical cancer?

A Once cervical cancer has progressed beyond carcinoma in situ, a hysterectomy and sometimes radiation therapy may be necessary. Some women will decide to have a hysterectomy if dysplasia or carcinoma in situ recurs or if they experience other gynecological problems with fibroids or irregular bleeding in addition to the precancerous changes or carcinoma in situ.

263

Q What is cervicitis?

A Cervicitis indicates an infection or inflammation of the cervix. This is not related to a precancerous change and is often not symptomatic. A chlamydia infection can cause cervicitis, but sometimes the cause cannot be determined.

264

Q What is the normal position of the uterus?

A The uterus is about the size of a woman's clenched fist and most commonly bends over the top of the bladder so that the top, or fundus, points toward the anterior abdominal wall. Because the uterus is so near the bladder in this position, the growth of the uterus in early pregnancy puts pressure on the bladder, causing the woman to feel as if she needs to urinate frequently.

265

Q Is it common to have a uterus that tips backward?

A A "tipped" uterus bends backward toward the rectum rather than over the bladder. This is a variant of normal and does not increase the incidence of infertility.

266

Q What is a fibroid tumor?

A Fibroids, also called myomas, are benign, smooth muscle tumors that most commonly occur in the uterus. Rarely they will grow in the smooth muscle layer of the esophagus, stomach, small intestine, large intestine, or rectum. Fibroids of the uterus are categorized according to their location in the uterine muscle. A subserous fibroid is found in the outer layer and protrudes outward into the abdominal cavity; an intramural fibroid is buried within the muscle layer of the uterus; and a submucous fibroid projects into the inside of the uterus. The submucous fibroid is most likely to cause heavy menses.

267

Q What should be done if the doctor finds fibroids?

A No therapy is necessary if a woman has not experienced any problems and the fibroids are discovered during a routine pelvic examination. Treatment may be needed if a woman has excessive bleeding, pain, infertility problems, or the fibroid is growing rapidly. Ultrasound evaluations can measure the size of the fibroid and the exact location.

268

Q How are fibroids diagnosed?

A A gynecologist or other health-care provider may feel the fibroids during a routine yearly pelvic examination.

Because a submucosal fibroid is likely to cause excessive bleeding and less likely to be felt during an exam, a pelvic sonogram may be ordered if a woman is having heavy periods. The sonogram is risk free, painless, and extremely accurate for the diagnosis of fibroids. Fibroids are occasionally diagnosed at a laparoscopy or other exploratory surgery.

269

Q Is a fibroid precancerous?

A Fibroids are slow growing and considered noncancerous because 99.9 percent are benign. The rare malignant fibroid grows rapidly.

270

Q Is there a way to remove the fibroids without removing the uterus in case the woman wants to have another child?

A A myomectomy is a procedure to remove fibroids without removing the uterus. This type of surgery is performed to remove enlarged or symptomatic fibroids in a woman who wishes to preserve her uterus.

271

Q Are there any medications to shrink fibroids?

A Depo-Lupron is a medication that is injected into a muscle every four weeks to significantly decrease the size of a uterine fibroid. A new injection that lasts three months is also now available. The fibroids will return once the injections are stopped. The woman taking the drug will experience menopausal symptoms such as hot flushes and dry vaginal tissues. The drug is not recommended for long-term treatment because of the risk of osteoporosis but is helpful in shrinking large fibroids in preparation for surgery.

272

Q What does it really mean when the doctor says your uterus is falling out?

A Sometimes after pregnancy and childbirth, the ligaments that support the uterus become stretched and the uterus falls from its natural position down into the vagina. This is called uterine descensus. If the descensus is mild, the patient may not have any symptoms, and no treatment is necessary. In some women, however, the problem can be so severe that the position of the uterus causes pain, difficulty with intercourse, and can actually come out of the vagina. There is a surgical procedure to resuspend the uterus into a normal position. This can be a difficult surgical procedure and should only be done by a doctor with significant experience in this specific type of surgery. If the woman doesn't desire future fertility, a hysterectomy is the best choice of treatment.

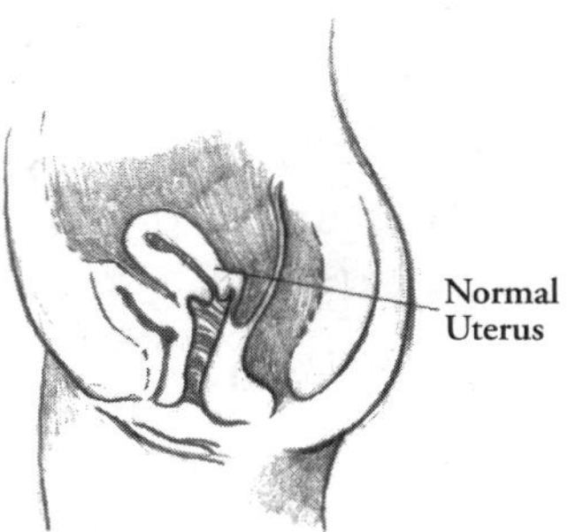

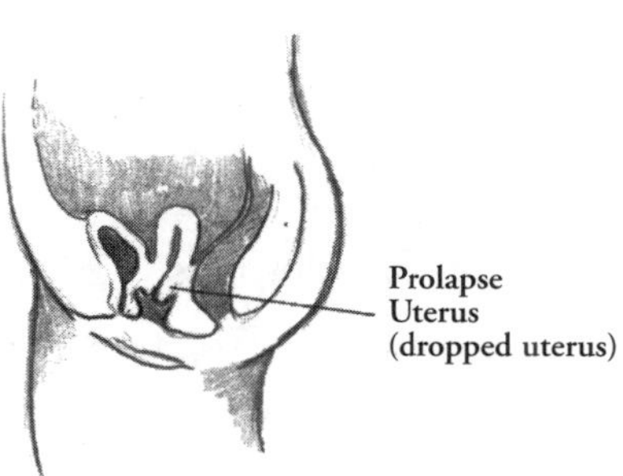

273

Q What is the uterus?

A The uterus is a hollow organ composed of several layers of smooth muscle. It is about the size of a woman's clenched fist and is located in the middle of the lower abdomen behind and just above the pubic bone. The mouth of the uterus, called the cervix, projects into the vagina, which communicates with the outside of the woman's body. In a mature woman, the lining of the uterus, called the endometrium, grows each month to prepare for the possible implantation of an embryo. If the woman doesn't become pregnant, the lining is shed causing the menstrual period. Blood and a small amount of tissue pass through the cervix, into the vagina, and then outside the body.

274

Q Do all women have a uterus?

A Although it's rare, there are women who have normal ovaries but are born without a uterus. Since these women have normal ovaries, they have normal female hormones, don't need any hormone replacement therapy, and will go through menopause at the natural time. The only way they can conceive a child is through in vitro fertilization and embryo implantation into a surrogate female.

275

Q Can a woman have two uteruses?

A The correct medical term for this condition is uterus didelphys. The uterus is formed in two parts that later fuse together in the midline of the developing female embryo body to form a single uterus. If this fusion fails to occur, two uteruses may be formed, each connected to one Fallopian tube with its ovary. Therefore, the woman will have two normal ovaries and tubes and two separate uteruses. Most of the time she can become pregnant in either uterus and successfully carry a pregnancy to maturity. It is necessary for these women to have two Pap smears each year at their annual checkup.

276

Q Is a uterine polyp cause for concern?

A Polyps are benign finger-like growths that are often found inside the uterus or the cervix. It is rare for them to have any malignant potential. They can sometimes be detected on a routine ultrasound procedure or during a dilatation and curettage (D and C) done for another reason. Polyps can cause irregular bleeding or spotting and can sometimes interfere with a woman's ability to get pregnant. Depending on the size of the polyp, the age of the woman, and her symptoms, the doctor may suggest that it be removed.

277

Q What is uterine cancer?

A Uterine cancer is found on the lining of the uterus (endometrium). Endometrial carcinoma found in its early stages is curable with a simple hysterectomy. This type of cancer more frequently occurs in women after the age of menopause.

278

Q What are the risk factors for uterine cancer?

A Women who have had normal, regular menstrual cycles are at low risk for uterine cancer until after menopause. High-risk women are those who have a hormone imbalance such as with polycystic ovaries. Irregular or infrequent cycles, obesity, diabetes, and high blood pressure are all known risk factors for endometrial carcinoma.

279

Q How can you prevent uterine cancer?

A Premenopausal women who have a problem with irregular or infrequent menstrual cycles due to a hormone imbalance should see their health-care provider. Using a form of progesterone or oral contraceptives will regulate a woman's monthly cycle and reduce her risk of uterine cancer.

280

Q How is uterine cancer treated?

A Early forms of endometrial cancer can be treated with a hysterectomy and removal of both tubes and ovaries without radiation therapy. More advanced stages require both surgery and radiation therapy. Chemotherapy is available to slow the growth of cancer cells in severe disease that has spread. Don't ignore irregular bleeding or other problems, especially after menopause. Early detection is important because endometrial cancer can be cured if found early.

281

Q What is a laparoscopy?

A This type of surgery allows the evaluation and treatment of pelvic and abdominal disease without making a large incision in a woman's body. A lens system much like a small telescope is placed into the abdominal cavity, often through an incision in the umbilicus (belly button). Carbon dioxide gas is pumped into the cavity to produce a large bubble or dome of gas that pushes

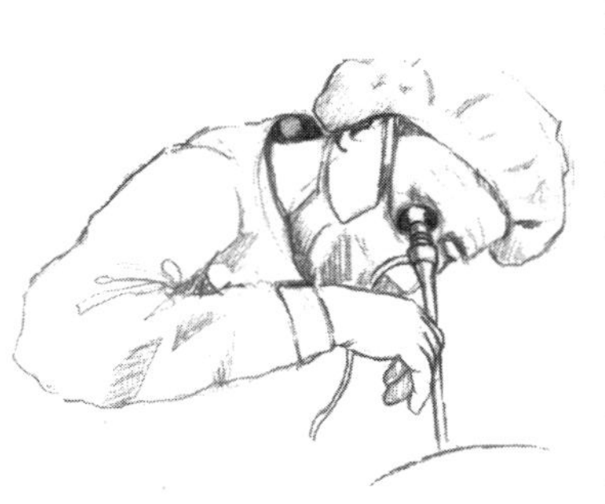

the intestines out of the way and allows the surgeon to clearly see the individual organs. Mini cameras now project the image from the laparoscope onto a television screen, and the entire surgery team can see and assist the operating surgeon. More than 50 percent of surgeries that used to require a major incision are now done using this procedure.

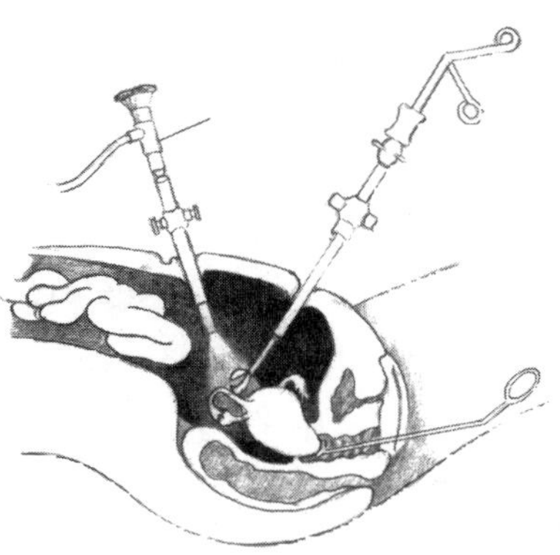

282

Q What is a hysterectomy?

A A hysterectomy is a surgical procedure in which the uterus is removed. A total hysterectomy means that the entire uterus including the cervix, which projects into the vagina, is removed. If a woman has a partial hysterectomy, the body of the uterus but not the cervix is removed. Some people feel the cervix provides some sensation during intercourse and should be preserved to maintain full sexual pleasure. The main sensation of pleasure during intercourse, however, is from the clitoris, which is not altered by a hysterectomy.

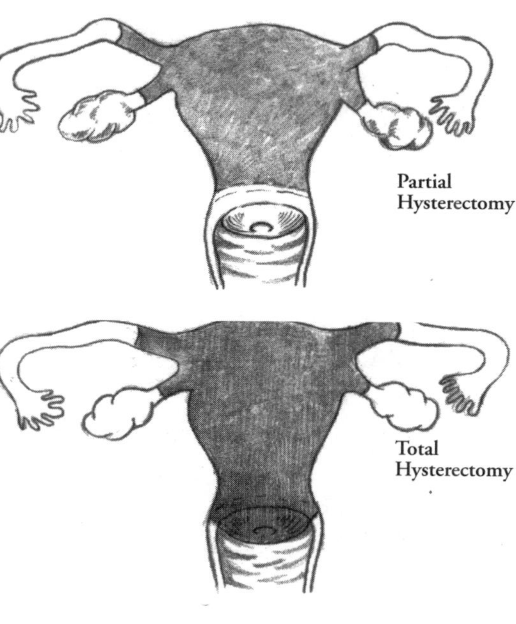

283

Q Why do different people need different types of hysterectomies?

A There are several different surgical options for performing a hysterectomy. Each has advantages and disadvantages. The traditional hysterectomy was done through a vertical incision from about the bottom of the umbilicus, or belly button, to the top of the pubic bone. In order to avoid a painful abdominal incision, the surgeon may do a vaginal hysterectomy where the uterus is removed through a vaginal incision.

284

Q What is the recovery time for a hysterectomy?

A All hysterectomies are considered major surgery. The surgery is basically the same regardless of the approach taken by the surgeon. Even though there is less pain from a vaginal hysterectomy, the vaginal incision as well as the internal surgery site needs to heal. Most surgeons suggest four to six weeks before full activity can be resumed.

285

Q Why can't a woman have intercourse until six weeks after having a hysterectomy?

A A seam is sutured at the back of the vagina after the cervix is removed during a hysterectomy. If you have intercourse before the area is healed, it could pop open and cause major complications. Nothing should be inserted into the vagina. Although you may have a slight discharge from healing, don't douche or use any vaginal products. Straining or lifting anything over five pounds might also damage the healing areas.

286

Q How soon can a woman go back to running and weight lifting after a hysterectomy?

A Women can walk without assistance when they leave the hospital. Start gradually increasing the distance walked and the speed. Walking outside is permitted within two weeks of the surgery. It's important to listen to your body and rest frequently. Slowly walking on a treadmill or stepper can usually be started by the end of the first four weeks. Do not do any significant weight lifting, abdominal exercises, or running until it has been cleared with the surgeon about six weeks after surgery.

287

Q Are the ovaries removed during a hysterectomy?

A The ovaries may or may not be removed during a hysterectomy. There is no reason to remove normal ovarian tissue if the reason for surgery is confined to the uterus.

288

Q Does bleeding between periods indicate a problem?

A Young women before menopause may normally have light bleeding or bloody mucus in the middle of a cycle about the time of egg release. Hormonal changes of perimenopause frequently cause erratic, unusual bleeding patterns. It's important that any persistent change, especially any unusual or unexpected bleeding during perimenopause or menopause, be investigated thoroughly. Cancer can cause the same symptoms.

289

Q What is endometriosis?

A Endometriosis is a common, benign disorder in which cells that normally line the uterus (endometrium) migrate to other parts of the body. Some women with this disease don't experience any pain. Others have debilitating, chronic pelvic pain, severe menstrual cramps, and pain with intercourse (dysparunia). The most common places for endometriosis to occur are the ovaries, the area between the uterus and the rectum, and the lining of the abdomen called the peritoneum. Less commonly, implants can occur on the bladder, intestines, and appendix. In rare instances, endometriosis will be found in the nose causing nose bleeds that coincide with the monthly menses. Endometriosis is a common cause of infertility.

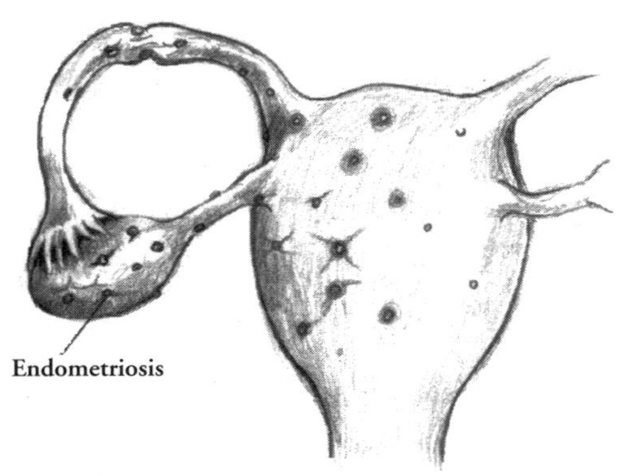

290

Q What causes endometriosis?

A Although the medical field theorizes the problem may be an immunological disorder, no one really knows the cause. About 90 percent of women have some menstrual fluid flow out of their Fallopian tubes into the abdominal cavity. The white blood cells in the abdominal cavity in most women "clean up" the blood and endometrial cells that get into the abdomen. In some women who develop endometriosis, the white cells and the immune system apparently don't destroy these cells and they are allowed to grow.

291

Q Can a woman expect to get endometriosis if her mother had it?

A Endometriosis does run in families. There is a seven times greater risk of getting endometriosis if a mother or sister has had it. The use of oral contraceptives may decrease the chance of getting endometriosis.

292

Q How is endometriosis diagnosed?

A A physician will perform a pelvic examination to try to detect abnormal tenderness, signs of scarring, or masses in the pelvis. A vaginal ultrasound is good at detecting cysts of endometriosis, called endometriomas, which can form inside the ovaries, but it is not sensitive enough to detect the small implants of endometriosis. By actually visualizing the abdomen and pelvic organs through a laparoscopy procedure, an accurate diagnosis and treatment of endometriosis can be made.

293

Q Once a woman has been treated for endometriosis is she cured?

A Endometriosis tends to be a recurrent disease. It is often necessary to treat the disease every eighteen to twenty-four months. Some women have more aggressive disease than others. Each woman has to be individually monitored for recurrence by her physician.

294

Q Does taking birth control pills help endometriosis?

A There are several ways to effectively treat endometriosis once a diagnosis is made. Taking oral contraceptives either in a regular, cyclical pattern or continuously (not taking the placebo) is a good way to partially suppress endometriosis. There are few side effects, and the birth control pills are relatively safe. This course of treatment is not effective for aggressive disease.

295

Q What is the injection that helps endometriosis?

A Depo-Lupron is a medication that is injected into a muscle every four weeks. A new form of Depo-Lupron, which is injected every three months, is now available as well. Because this drug causes a temporary menopause, estrogen levels drop very low and the implants of endometriosis, which are hormonally responsive, begin to "dry up." The menopause symptoms of hot flushes, dry vaginal tissues, and decreased breast size are reversed when the medication is discontinued. This medication is not intended for long-term use because of the risk of premature osteoporosis.

296

Q If a woman is having difficulty getting pregnant, could it have anything to do with being treated for endometriosis in the past?

A Although endometriosis can cause infertility, it is wise to have a basic fertility evaluation to be certain that nothing else is wrong. A woman should probably have another laparoscopy to evaluate her endometriosis, treat any active implants, and remove adhesions that might be decreasing her chance of pregnancy.

297

Q What hormones are produced by the ovaries?

A The two ovaries contain egg units that produce the two female hormones estrogen and progesterone. They also produce a small amount of the male hormone testosterone.

298

Q What is polycystic ovarian disease?

A This is a hormonal disorder characterized by irregular menstrual cycles, increased production of male hormone, oily skin, acne, infertility due to irregular ovulation, and an increased risk of obesity. Because of the irregular or infrequent cycles, these patients are at increased risk of uterine cancer as they get older. They also have a higher incidence of adult onset diabetes.

299

Q What causes ovarian cysts?

A There are a variety of types of ovarian cysts. The most common type is called a simple cyst and may be an egg unit that failed to rupture on schedule. Instead of opening to release the egg, fluid continues to build up in the follicle to form a large fluid-filled sac. Oral contraceptives help decrease the chance of having an ovarian cyst.

300

Q How are ovarian cysts treated?

A Some ovarian cysts resolve without treatment. If the woman is not experiencing a great deal of pain, the most common treatment would be for her to take oral contraceptives for one month. The cyst will often resolve itself without surgery. If the pill is not successful, a laparoscopy to remove or drain a persistent cyst may be necessary.

301

Q Will a woman have difficulty getting pregnant if one of her ovaries has been removed?

A It takes one healthy ovary and tube on the same side for pregnancy. One ovary contains enough healthy eggs for a woman to have any number of children.

302

Q What are the risk factors for ovarian cancer?

A Ovarian cancer is a silent and deadly type of cancer. The average woman has a 1.3 percent risk of having ovarian cancer in her lifetime. Less than 7 percent of women who have ovarian cancer have a family history. A woman whose mother or sister has had it is at a slightly increased risk because some families have a genetically inherited high risk for ovarian cancer. Women who have been pregnant or take oral contraceptives have a decreased risk. It is important to have regular pelvic examinations by a physician.

303

Q How can a woman protect herself against ovarian cancer?

A The best protection is to take oral contraceptives. The risk of ovarian cancer is decreased by 80 percent if the pill has been taken for at least eight years.

304

Q Why do some women have to urinate so frequently?

A Some women urinate a lot because they have low bladder capacity and can only hold a small amount of fluid. Others can have an irritable bladder that contracts before the woman wishes to urinate. Women who drink a lot of water will urinate frequently.

Keeping a diary of fluid intake for twenty-four hours and measuring urinary output will help the physician determine what might be causing the problem.

305

Q Why do women have so many urinary track infections?

A The urethra, which leads from the bladder to outside, is very short in a woman. Bacteria from the vagina or from intercourse can be rubbed into the urethra and make its way into the bladder. This is one reason it's important to wipe from front to back after urinating or having a bowel movement, to minimize the risk of moving bacteria from vagina or rectum toward the urethra. Urinating after intercourse may also be helpful.

306

Q What can be done to help prevent bladder infections?

A Several steps can be taken to help in the prevention of bladder infections. It's important to urinate when you feel the urge, wipe from front to back after urinating or having a bowel movement to avoid moving bacteria from the vagina or rectum toward the urethra, drink six to eight glasses of water a day, and urinate after sexual relations to remove any of the bacteria that may have entered the urethra. Some women take an antibiotic after intercourse to suppress a bladder infection.

307

Q What is incontinence?

A Incontinence is the loss of urine to the outside of the body when it's not intended. Although accidental loss of urine doesn't harm a woman's health, it can be a major source of embarrassment. The female is more likely to be incontinent because her urethra is so much shorter than the male urethra.

308

Q Is there anything a woman can do to prevent the loss of urine when she coughs or sneezes?

A When pressure is introduced into the abdominal cavity from a cough or sneeze, a spurt of urine may be lost from the bladder. Losing urine in this way is called stress incontinence. Although surgery may be necessary in some cases to restore the natural anatomy of the bladder and urethra, strengthening the pelvic floor muscles with Kegel exercises can sometimes help.

309

Q How are Kegel exercises done?

A Kegel exercises are done to strengthen the muscles that support the pelvic organs, including the bladder and vagina. Increased control of the pubococcygeus muscle allows a woman to have better control of urination and may increase sexual satisfaction.

It can be difficult for a woman to learn how to contract this muscle. A good way to start is to place two fingers into the vagina and practice squeezing your fingers with the vaginal muscle. To do Kegels, contract these muscles, hold for a count of three, and then relax. Start out with ten contractions at a time, and add five a week until you can do twenty-five in a row. Try to do at least five sets each day. Vary the exercise by doing quick, fast Kegels followed by a set of strong, slow contractions. You can do your Kegels at a stoplight or anywhere else you have a free moment. No one will even know you're doing them!

310

Q Why do some women have to get up several times during the night to go to the bathroom?

A Lying down improves the blood flow to the kidneys and the fluid that has accumulated in your legs during the day is released. To avoid the nighttime trips, try to limit salt intake, get regular exercise to stimulate good circulation, put your feet up during the day to limit fluid accumulation in the legs, and decrease fluids after 4:00 P.M.

311

Q Will surgery help a woman who is losing urine when she doesn't want to?

A Surgery may be needed if conservative treatments, such as physical therapy to strengthen the muscles of the pelvic floor, voiding frequently to decrease stress on the bladder, and controlling caffeine and fluid intakes, don't help. There are many different types of surgical procedures to help restore the normal position of the urethra and the bladder. It is important to have a surgeon who specializes in these types of surgery do the preoperative evaluation and the surgery. There is at most an 80 percent long-term success rate with this type of surgery.

312

Q Is there any help for a woman who can't even leave her house because by the time she realizes she has to urinate it's usually too late?

A Some women experience "urge incontinence" where they run to the bathroom as soon as they have the urge to urinate but it may be too late. Avoidance of caffeine, which irritates the bladder, and going to the bathroom regularly every hour whether it's necessary or not keeps the bladder from getting too full. Keeping a diary for twenty-four hours of fluid intake and measuring urinary output will help the physician decide what might be causing the problem. There are medications if the condition warrants it.

313

Q Is dark yellow urine a cause for concern?

A When a person is dehydrated, the urine has a dark color. The color will be diluted to a pale yellow when enough water is being consumed. Vitamin B will also change the urine to a dark yellow color.

314

Q Can a woman drink too much water?

A It's healthy to drink six to eight regular glasses of water a day. If more is consumed, the body will regulate itself by making more urine. The end result is spending a great deal of time urinating.

The Digestive Tract

315

Q What can a woman do for frequent constipation?

A Many women feel they are constipated if they don't have a bowel movement every day. It is normal, however, to have a bowel movement three times a week. Constipation can be controlled with a diet high in fresh fruits and vegetables, bran, raisins, prunes, figs, and whole grains. Gradually increase fiber into the diet to avoid bloating. Adequate fluid intake and exercise are also important.

316

Q How much fiber is enough?

A Adding too much fiber at one time will make the body become bloated and crampy. A woman shouldn't need more than forty grams (about an ounce) of a bulk stool softener like Metamucil daily added to a reasonable diet.

317

Q What can a woman do for painful hemorrhoids?

A Hemorrhoids are dilated veins found in the anus. They are more common in women during pregnancy. Although rarely dangerous, they can cause pain and swelling. It's important to avoid constipation because hard stools irritate the hemorrhoids causing increased pain. Gently pushing back a hemorrhoid that protrudes out of the anal opening may help relieve some pain. Sitting in a warm tub of water or applying petroleum jelly or witch hazel can also be soothing to the anal area. Although women report relief from over-the-counter hemorrhoid preparations, there is no scientific evidence that they work. If hemorrhoid problems are acute, the doctor may recommend they be surgically removed. Recovery includes several weeks of severe discomfort and pain until the area heals.

318

Q What should a woman do when she sees blood in her stool?

A Hemorrhoids are the most common cause of bright red rectal bleeding. More serious problems, including rectal cancer, may cause bleeding. Rectal bleeding should be evaluated by a physician. An X ray of the colon or having the area examined with a flexible lighted tube may be recommended.

319

Q Should a woman be concerned if her bowel movements seem to be getting much darker?

A The color of stool is usually determined by diet. More leafy green vegetables or taking a vitamin with iron will turn the stool a dark color. However, stools that are black, sticky, and foul smelling may be due to bleeding from the stomach or intestines. These findings should be reported to a physician immediately.

320

Q How can a woman with a family history of colon cancer protect herself?

A You are more likely to develop colon cancer if you are over forty years old, drink excessive amounts of alcohol (more than two drinks a day), experience constipation, or have a family history. A healthy diet, high in fiber and low in fat, can make a difference. A recent study showed that women who take four to six aspirin a week had a lower incidence of colon cancer. A colonoscopy is recommended for a woman at forty if she has a positive family history. If the test is clear, another is not necessary for five years.

321

Q What is a colonoscopy?

A A colonoscopy is a test that allows a physician to look into the large intestines. Before the test, the woman cleanses the colon by drinking a large quantity of a prescription laxative. Under sedation, the doctor will use a flexible lighted tube to check the colon for any abnormalities. A baseline test is recommended between ages forty and fifty and does not have to be repeated for five years unless an abnormality is found.

322

Q Is something wrong if a woman sometimes has diarrhea and is then constipated?

A Any change in bowel habits should be reported to the doctor. Usually alternating diarrhea and constipation are symptoms of irritable bowel syndrome. This is a common problem that stress appears to make worse. Laxatives or diarrhea medicines should not be taken. Increased fiber in the diet, regular exercise, and stress reduction techniques should be tried before considering prescribed medications.

323

Q How often should a woman have a bowel movement?

A There is a wide range of normalcy in the frequency of bowel movements. It is normal to have a bowel movement up to three times a day or as infrequently as three times a week.

324

Q Is there anything that can be done for weakness between the vagina and rectum?

A The tissue between the rectum and vagina can be stretched or traumatized by childbirth. A weakness in this area may cause a bulge into the vagina called a rectocoele. Some women have to place their fingers into the vagina (splinting) to have a normal bowel movement. Strengthening the muscles of the pelvic floor with Kegel exercises may help a little, but the main treatment is surgery. A surgeon can repair this defect and increase the strength of the vaginal-rectal wall.

325

Q Does taking laxatives on a regular basis cause any problems?

A Chronic use of laxatives causes the bowel to become laxative dependent so that it won't contract normally without the use of the laxative. Introducing a bulk or natural laxative such as psyllium will help the elimination process if adequate water is taken. Regular exercise such as walking encourages the intestine to contract properly. Talk to your doctor if you are laxative dependent or have other related problems.

326

Q What could be wrong with a woman who feels pain in the lower right side of her abdomen?

A There are many different organs that could cause pain in that area including the right ovary and tube, large and small intestines, the ureter (right tube from the kidney to the bladder), muscles, bones, and skin that form the abdomen. The bladder and uterus are in the midline at the bottom of the abdomen but may seem to hurt on the right side. The appendix, which is part of the bowel, is usually, but not always, on the right side.

327

Q What is the appendix?

A The appendix is a hollow finger-like projection off the large intestine. It doesn't seem to have an important function and can become infected and inflamed (appendicitis). If an infected appendix isn't treated promptly, it can rupture and spread infection from the bowel into the abdomen causing a serious and potentially fatal infection called peritonitis.

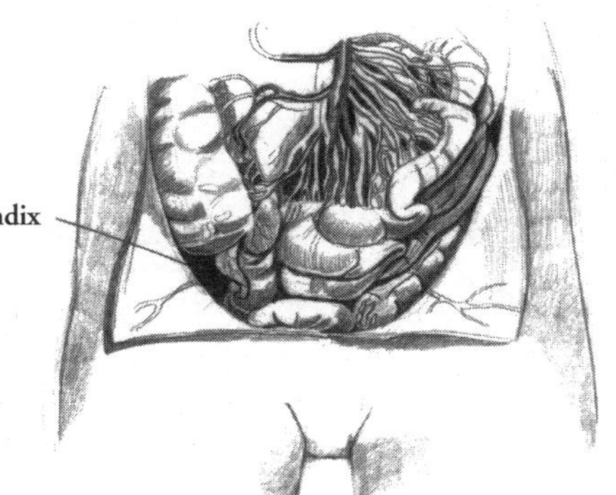

328

Q What are the symptoms of appendicitis?

A The major symptom of appendicitis is pain, which may start around the belly button (umbilicus) and then move over to the right lower quadrant of the abdomen. When a physician pushes on the abdomen over the inflamed appendix, the patient feels pain and tenderness. When the doctor lets go suddenly, the patient has intense pain called "rebound." The lining of the abdomen, the peritoneum, is inflamed by the developing infection. If the peritoneum is suddenly moved, it is very painful. In addition to pain, the patient with appendicitis often complains of nausea with or without vomiting, has a lack of appetite, and runs a fever. Sometimes appendicitis is "classical" in its symptoms and other times it's difficult to diagnosis.

329

Q Why can't an appendicitis infection be treated with antibiotics rather than surgery?

A The inside of the abdomen is sterile, meaning there isn't any bacteria. The inside of the large bowel is full of a variety of bacteria that help to digest the fecal material. The bowel wall protects the rest of the body from being infected with bacteria. If the appendix is infected and ruptures, releasing the bowel bacteria into the abdominal cavity, a life-threatening infection called peritonitis occurs. Surgery to remove the appendix is the only way to prevent the spread of bacteria.

330

Q If a woman has cramps and abdominal pain that seem to move from place to place, should she see a doctor?

A Cramps and abdominal pain are often caused by irritable bowel or functional bowel disease. Women with this problem tend to have constipation alternating with diarrhea or loose stools. Functional means that the anatomy of the bowel is normal. The contraction, or motility, of the bowel is abnormal. However, you can't necessarily distinguish irritable bowel, which is a benign disease, from early colon cancer or other bowel disorders without an evaluation. A colonoscopy is usually suggested to look inside the bowel.

331

Q Why do some women avoid wheat products?

A The internal lining of the small intestine is lined by microvilli, which are little projections that absorb food. In people with celiac disease, the gluten from wheat is toxic to the microvilli. When a woman eats gluten (bread, pasta, cereal), it doesn't get absorbed normally because the microvilli are destroyed. Avoiding wheat products is difficult but helps the woman to avoid illness.

332

Q What is ulcerative colitis?

A Ulcerative colitis is an inflammatory disease of the large intestine (colon). Women with this disorder have abdominal pain and diarrhea that may contain blood or pus. It is an autoimmune disorder with periods of exacerbation and spontaneous remission. Arthritis and skin rashes may occur. The disease is most often treated with anti-inflammatory medications. Patients with long-standing ulcerative colitis have a greater risk of colon cancer and should be checked by a physician regularly.

333

Q What is Crohn's disease?

A Crohn's disease is an inflammatory disease of the gastrointestinal tract. It can cause abdominal pain, diarrhea, poor appetite, weight loss, skin rashes, and joint pain. The diagnosis is made by X rays of the GI tract using barium and looking into the colon with a lighted, flexible tube (colonoscopy). Anti-inflammatory drugs are helpful in the control of the disease.

334

Q What is diverticulosis?

A A diverticulum is an out-pouching of the large bowel, which causes a pocket-like sac to form. These can become infected (diverticulitis) or rupture, causing abdominal pain. Antibiotics may be helpful in some cases while surgery may be required in others. Diagnosis is made using a colon X-ray or looking inside the colon with a lighted, flexible tube (colonoscopy).

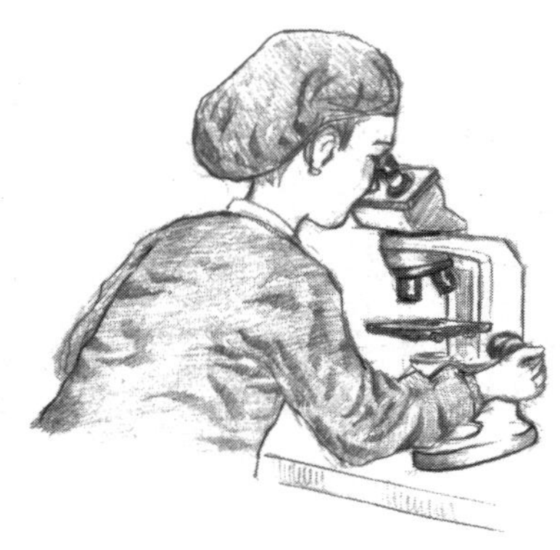

Sexuality and Sexually Transmitted Diseases

335

Q What is normal sexual behavior?

A Any sexual activity between consenting adults, which doesn't physically or mentally harm either, is considered to be normal.

336

Q How often is it normal to have sex?

A There are no "normal" values for frequency of sexual activity. Sometimes couples have conflicts because one partner wants to have sex more often than the other. Some couples are happy with once or twice a month while others have sex daily. Sexual desire (libido) seems to vary over time depending on daily stresses, health, and age. As long as you and your partner are happy with your sex life, it doesn't matter how often you have sex. On the other hand, if you can't agree on how often to have sex and this causes serious problems in your relationship, you should consider seeing a counselor.

337

Q Why would a woman who loves her partner not want to have sex?

A Love and sexual desire are not the same thing. A woman can experience deep feelings about someone but not want to participate in the physical sex act. If your lack of desire is harming your relationship, see your gynecologist for a physical exam. If she determines there is no physical cause, she can recommend a sexual therapist.

338

Q What is sexual preference?

A Some people desire a physical, sexual relationship with a person of the opposite sex (heterosexual) while others prefer same-sex relationships (homosexual). There is a continuum of sexual preference from purely heterosexual to purely homosexual. Many people repressed their homosexual feelings in the past because they were not accepted by mainstream society. It is normal, however, for heterosexual people to have some homosexual thoughts or desires.

339

Q Why does my husband want to videotape our sexual experiences?

A Although both sexes often enjoy seeing sexually explicit material, men seek this activity more than women. There is nothing wrong or deviant about taping personal sexual activity for personal use if both parties feel comfortable with the experience.

340

Q What is an orgasm?

A An orgasm is the culmination of a series of events that occur during a sexual experience. During the initial excitement, or arousal phase, heart rate increases and the vagina and clitoris become engorged with blood. The vaginal walls produce a slick, clear, lubricating fluid. As sexual excitement increases, the woman reaches a plateau phase, which is the peak of excitement and blood engorgement. When orgasm occurs, there is a release of tension followed by the resolution phase where the woman's body returns to its pre-excitement state.

341

Q Is there something wrong with a woman who has never had an orgasm?

A It is rare that a healthy woman can't reach orgasm. Sometimes women don't receive enough sexual stimulation to go through the phases of excitement and plateau to reach orgasm. Others, because of learned taboos, bad sexual experiences, or other psychological problems, aren't orgasmic. Many women enjoy sex without the orgasm. Women can often learn to be orgasmic by masturbation and then in a shared experience. A sex therapist is usually able to help a woman become orgasmic.

342

Q What is foreplay?

A Traditionally foreplay means stimulation to increase sexual excitement prior to vaginal-penile penetration in a heterosexual relationship. Foreplay can include almost any type of stimulation: seeing a partner, hearing words of affection, odors, fantasies, music, and physical touch.

343

Q What is the clitoris?

A The clitoris is a small area of erectile tissue located at the top of the labia, which surround the female genital opening. It is just above the urethral opening where urine comes out and is covered by a hood of tissue. The clitoris is derived from the same tissue as the glans at the end of the male penis. It is extremely sensitive to the touch. Stimulating the clitoris directly or indirectly causes intense pleasure for most women.

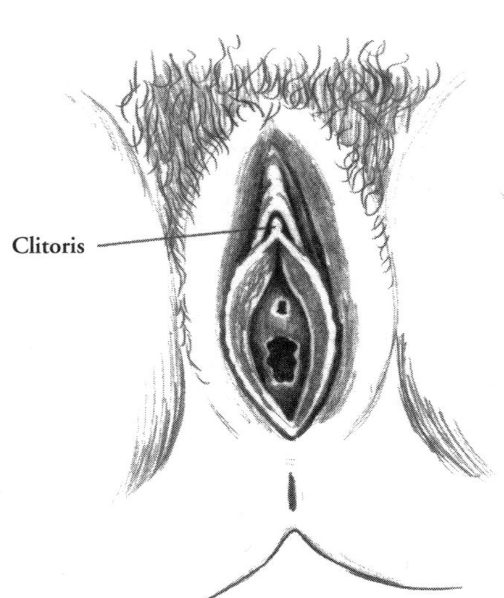

344

Q Is there a difference in clitoral and vaginal orgasms?

A Sigmund Freud suggested there were two different types of orgasms. An orgasm caused by vaginal intercourse was supposed to be better and more mature than an orgasm caused manually or by oral stimulation of the clitoris. What Freud considered a vaginal orgasm occurred during penile penetration, but its cause is the clitoris being stimulated by the hood as the penis moves the vaginal lips. Therefore, there is really only one type of orgasm: clitoral.

345

Q What is the G spot?

A Research has not been able to verify a specific spot on the front wall of the vagina called the G spot. Although a woman may identify sexual pleasure with stimulation from many areas of the body, most genital sexual sensation is related to stimulation of the clitoris.

346

Q Why would a woman's sexual fantasies include violence?

A Many women have sexual fantasies about other people or other types of sexual activity than they typically engage in. Sometimes these fantasies include unusual or violent behavior. Experiencing a fantasy doesn't mean the woman wants to participate in the activity. These fantasies are not harmful unless they interfere with a woman's life in a destructive way.

347

Q What can a woman do to escalate her sexual desire if it has diminished since giving birth?

A Rarely does childbirth physically alter the ability of a woman to be sexually responsive. However, the responsibilities of a new baby and adjusting to new routines can leave a woman with little time or energy for sex. In addition, some women feel less desirable until they regain their body shape. Lack of sexual desire can be a symptom of depression, which is not uncommon in the postpartum months. These problems usually correct themselves with time and patience, but if your life is not getting back to normal two to three months after the birth of a baby, seek the help of a counselor.

348

Q Can taking antidepressants decrease sexual desire?

A Some antidepressants, such as Prozac, Paxil, and Zoloft, can decrease sexual desire. Sometimes it is difficult to determine whether the medication or the depression itself is the cause of sexual dysfunction. Discuss your concerns with your health-care provider, who may suggest you try other medications.

349

Q Why does a woman's body image sometimes affect her interest in sex?

A For many women it's important to feel good about their body before they are comfortable sharing it with someone else. This feeling may not have anything to do with the partner's attitude at all. It's important to share these concerns with a partner to achieve an intimate relationship. Also, keeping in good physical shape, which does not mean you have to look like Miss America, makes everyone feel better.

350

Q Why is it sometimes difficult for women to have sex with their partners when they're angry or don't feel loved?

A Emotions are an important part of human sexuality. Any upsetting emotion, such as anger, grief, depression, or anxiety, will often affect the sex drive. It's important to share your feelings with your partner to achieve an intimate relationship. It may be helpful to talk with a therapist if these episodes occur on a regular basis.

351

Q Is pornography dangerous?

A Although there is little data to suggest pornography is dangerous, everyone agrees it should be restricted to consenting adults. Many healthy, well-adjusted people enjoy pornographic magazines and X-rated movies. Although there is much controversy over what types of sexual activity are unacceptable and over interference with freedom of speech, child pornography is both culturally condemned and illegal.

352

Q Is it normal for a female to masturbate?

A Masturbation is normal, and young girls will do it unless they are told it is bad or abnormal. It is the best way for a woman to learn to be sexually responsive and orgasmic. Once a woman teaches herself what is most pleasurable, she will be able to instruct her partner. Masturbation is achieved most often by a woman rubbing her clitoris with her fingers.

353

Q How should a woman handle a partner who is pressuring her to have sex when she isn't ready?

A If one partner feels that the success of the relationship depends solely on sexual intimacy, there is a serious problem. A woman should not participate in a sexual relationship until she is a willing partner. A loving partner will understand that a woman may not be ready to have sex but still cares about him.

354

Q Can a doctor tell if a woman is a virgin?

A Most of the time even a gynecologist cannot be certain whether a woman has been sexually active or not. Some women have a thick ring of tissue, the hymen, that has to be stretched by the penis to gain entry into the vagina. This stretching can cause discomfort and sometimes bleeding. The ring may be so thick that the hymen has to be removed by a doctor prior to successful intercourse. The hymen is thin and flexible, most often permitting intercourse without trauma.

355

Q Can a woman's partner tell if she's a virgin?

A It's unlikely that a partner could tell whether a woman is a virgin or not because the opening of the vagina before any sexual activity varies from one woman to another. A tight vaginal opening may suggest a woman has not been sexually active, but this is not always the case. Similarly, a large vaginal opening does not indicate a woman has had intercourse.

356

Q Does intercourse always hurt the first time?

A Some women have no pain with their first intercourse while others may experience a burning sensation and perhaps a small amount of bleeding. In order to produce adequate lubrication of the vagina, it is important for the woman to have plenty of sexual stimulation prior to attempting vaginal penetration. A visit with a health-care provider prior to intercourse will determine if there are any problems that would make a first-time experience difficult.

357

Q Is it better to have intercourse in a certain position?

A Position for intercourse or any other sexual activity is strictly a matter of personal preference. The idea that the missionary position is better has no scientific basis. In fact, many couples prefer the female superior position so that she can control her stimulation better. Couples should experiment with different ways of sexual gratification to enrich their sexual experience.

358

Q What can a woman do if her partner has trouble getting an erection?

A There are medical illnesses, such as diabetes, and medications, such as antidepressants and antihypertensives, that interfere with erections. Both men and women need increased stimulation as they get older to achieve sexual excitement. The female may need to offer increased foreplay such as oral or manual penile stimulation. Medications that can improve erection are available, so a urologist should be consulted if the problem persists.

359

Q If a woman's partner can't get an erection, is it because something is wrong with her?

A Erectile dysfunction can occur for a variety of reasons that have no bearing on the partner. A woman can only try to relax her partner and offer increased penile stimulation. She is not equipped, however, to resolve his issue if a medical illness or psychological problem exists.

360

Q Where is information available about new medications for men who have trouble getting erections?

A A urologist or family physician would be a good source of information. Several sexual aids are available, including rings, suction devices, and a new soft gel that can be placed into the tip of the penis to stimulate blood flow and help to maintain erection.

361

Q Will a hysterectomy affect a woman's sex life?

A Most women don't notice any difference sexually after a hysterectomy because it doesn't alter the clitoris, which accounts for most of the pleasure during sexual activity. Some women report increased pleasure from knowing they don't have to be concerned about birth control. There are also reports of improvement in sexual activity because the woman is no longer uncomfortable from bleeding or pelvic pain.

362

Q Should couples always have simultaneous orgasms?

A Most sex therapists feel it's unrealistic for a couple to have simultaneous orgasms on a regular basis. The female, in a heterosexual relationship, often requires more stimulation than her male partner. Many couples concentrate on stimulating the woman to orgasm and then the man. It is important for the couple to talk with and satisfy each other.

363

Q Is there something wrong with a woman who can't have an orgasm through intercourse alone?

A Actually, 30 to 40 percent of women cannot achieve orgasm with only intercourse. They may require oral or manual stimulation or the use of a vibrator. Some can only be orgasmic with masturbation. It is normal for a woman to need more clitoral stimulation in addition to intercourse to accomplish an orgasm.

364

Q What exactly does sadomasochism mean?

A Sadomasochism, or S&M, is a controversial type of sexual relationship. One partner has their sexual satisfaction increased by inflicting pain on another person (sadism). The other partner has increased sexual satisfaction from experiencing pain or humiliation (masochism). Most sex therapists think that mild forms of this relationship fall within the range of acceptable behavior. Both partners, however, must agree to the activity and neither should be harmed by it. There is a fine line between abuse and acceptability. A woman should seek counseling if she feels she is in a destructive relationship.

365

Q What does having AIDS really mean?

A AIDS is caused by an infection with a virus called human immunodeficiency virus, or HIV. This virus can attack the immune system, making the person more susceptible to infections. Not all people who test positive for HIV are ill. It may take years for the infection to show symptoms.

366

Q How do people get AIDS?

A AIDS is spread by sharing body fluids. The highest risk activities are intravenous drug use and anal intercourse. During anal intercourse, there are often rectal tears, which allow entry of the AIDS virus infected cells. During heterosexual intercourse, females are more likely to be infected by males than the other way around. This virus can also be transmitted through the placenta from the mother to her child. Transmission of the virus by lesbian partners is rare. AIDS can also be acquired through blood transfusions or blood products, although today's blood supply is considered safe.

367

Q Why should women worry about AIDS if it's mainly a disease of homosexual males?

A AIDS is not just a disease of homosexual males. The highest risk group are intravenous drug abusers followed by homosexual men. However, women are acquiring AIDS faster than any other group in the United States and are being infected by heterosexual intercourse. Women should protect themselves by using condoms during intercourse unless they are in a long-term, mutually exclusive, monogamous relationship.

368

Q Is it dangerous to shake hands or hug someone with AIDS?

A Casual physical contact does not transmit the AIDS virus. There is no reason to be afraid of skin-to-skin contact such as hugging or shaking hands. Kissing is a low-risk activity unless there are sores in the mouth or on the lips. The AIDS virus finds its way into the body through a scratch, sore, or cut. There is no danger working or going to school with an HIV-positive person.

369

Q What are the symptoms of AIDS?

A The symptoms can be very nonspecific, such as fatigue, swollen lymph nodes, a cough, diarrhea, swollen joints, skin rash, poor coordination, and unexplained fever. In some parts of Africa, AIDS is called "thin disease" because the patients often have rapid weight loss. Women with AIDS have more frequent and severe vaginal yeast infections. There is also a higher incidence of abnormal Pap smears and cervical cancer in women who are infected. All areas of the body become more susceptible to infections as the immune system gets weaker.

370

Q Should I get tested if I think I might have been exposed to AIDS?

A Early diagnosis has become very important because of the increased success of medical therapy to control the symptoms and disease progression. An AIDS test should always be done before a woman becomes pregnant to keep the unborn child from risk. There are a number of ways to be tested anonymously. Contact a local AIDS support group for more information about services in your area.

371

Q Should I be tested for AIDS if I'm already pregnant?

A There are new medical studies that suggest a decrease in the chance of a baby getting AIDS from an infected mother if she is given medication during pregnancy. If you are pregnant you should get an AIDS test. It may save your baby's life.

372

Q How soon can I get a blood test after exposure to the virus?

A One to three months after possible exposure is a good baseline reading. However, the test should be repeated three months after that.

373

Q How can I decrease my chances of getting AIDS?

A A woman should avoid blood transfusions unless it's absolutely necessary, avoid intravenous drugs, limit sexual partners, and use condoms until a relationship has been mutually monogamous for at least three years. Foam vaginal contraceptives may help decrease AIDS transmission but don't work as well as latex condoms. The birth control pill does not prevent AIDS.

374

Q What treatments are available for AIDS?

A Some medications are available to help improve the immune system while others suppress the virus. Infections need to be aggressively treated when they occur. New drugs and drug combinations are being improved constantly to give hope of remission or eradication.

375

Q How could I be infected with pubic lice if I haven't had intercourse with anyone in months?

A Pubic lice, crabs, are transmitted by close personal contact. However, this problem can also be caused by contact with infected linens or clothing. Although they don't pose a serious health threat, pubic lice cause severe itching.

376

Q How are pubic lice treated?

A It is important to wash all linens and underclothes in hot water and have them thoroughly dried. Items that can't be washed should be sprayed with a special antiseptic solution or sealed in a plastic bag for at least two weeks to allow the lice to die. There are several effective over-the-counter treatments for pubic lice that your pharmacist can recommend.

377

Q What causes genital warts?

A Genital warts are caused by a highly contagious papilloma virus. Some forms of the virus are associated with precancerous or cancerous lesions of the cervix. Warts can be transmitted from other areas of the body but are usually transmitted by sexual contact. Some warts are large and bulky while others are microscopic in size.

378

Q Do condoms help protect women from genital warts?

A Condoms offer some protection from contracting the papilloma virus. There can be small, microscopic warts, however, on the male scrotum, which isn't covered by the male condom. The female condom may be somewhat more protective since it covers the external female genitalia. Sometimes the warts are so small the male doesn't notice them and doesn't realize he is putting his partner at risk.

379

Q How are genital warts treated?

A Large warts are usually removed surgically while small ones are treated with a caustic solution, a laser, or frozen. The male partners of women with warts should be checked by a urologist to see if they may be carrying the virus. It is difficult, if not impossible, for the virus to be completely eradicated.

380

Q How would a woman know if she had a chlamydia infection?

A If a woman is sexually active and not in a long-term, mutually monogamous relationship, she should have a chlamydia test done at the same time as the yearly Pap smear. Persistent lower abdominal pain and tenderness may indicate chlamydia.

381

Q Can chlamydia be prevented?

A The risk of chlamydia is decreased, as with all STDs, by limiting sexual partners, knowing their sexual history, and using latex condoms. A male may not even experience any symptoms of the disease.

382

Q How is chlamydia treated?

A Chlamydia is susceptible to certain antibiotics, such as doxycycline. You need to take all of your medication and have a follow-up test to make sure the treatment worked. Sometimes a second course of antibiotics is needed. It is also important for a woman's sexual partner(s) to be tested and treated.

383

Q Is gonorrhea still a common STD?

A Gonorrhea, sometimes known as "the clap," is the second most common sexually transmitted disease in the United States and is responsible for 30 to 40 percent of cases of pelvic inflammatory disease. Many women have no symptoms while men can experience a thick penile discharge and pain with urination.

384

Q How is gonorrhea detected?

A A diagnosis of gonorrhea is made by culturing the organism from the body fluids, usually from the cervix. Because there may be no symptoms in women, and because it can cause serious pelvic infections, a woman at risk should be screened yearly. An immediate evaluation is necessary for persistent pelvic pain, tenderness, or abnormal vaginal discharge.

385

Q How is gonorrhea treated?

A Gonorrhea is quickly eradicated by penicillin therapy, which is readily available and inexpensive. People with penicillin allergies can take doxycycline. Some physicians prefer using doxycycline since people with gonorrhea are also at risk for chlamydia infections, which don't respond to penicillin. There have been some resistant strains of gonorrhea, so follow-up cultures should always be done. It's important that all sexual partners be tested and treated if found to have the disease.

386

Q Can a woman get gonorrhea or other sexually transmitted disease by having oral sex?

A Most sexually transmitted diseases, including gonorrhea, can be transmitted by oral, anal, or vaginal contact.

387

Q Can a woman contract a sexually transmitted disease if the man doesn't ejaculate?

A Most sexually transmitted diseases, including AIDS, can be transmitted whether the man ejaculates or not. Withdrawal is not adequate for prevention of infection. Use of latex condoms anytime there is penile-vaginal contact is imperative for disease prevention.

388

Q How can a person get hepatitis from sexual contact?

A Hepatitis B is a viral disease that causes inflammation of the liver and is often spread by sexual contact. It is extremely infectious and can be passed through any body fluid. Some people may have a mild form of the disease with fever, tiredness, muscle aches, and low-grade fever while others become very ill and turn yellow (jaundice). Most recover but about 5 percent experience chronic liver inflammation.

There is no way to treat hepatitis B, but the new vaccine, which can prevent the spread of the organism, is recommended.

389

Q Is a woman likely to get a genital herpes virus infection if she gets recurrent fever blisters?

A Historically, Type I herpes caused fever blisters and Type II caused genital blisters. It is now understood that both types can affect the mouth and the genital tissues. Fever blisters don't increase the risk of genital herpes as long as the woman practices careful hygiene. You should wash your hands after touching a fever blister and before touching the genital organs to avoid transmission.

390

Q What symptoms does a herpes infection cause?

A A woman may experience flulike symptoms with fever and muscle aches if it's her first exposure to the virus. The first outbreak of the typical blisterlike lesions may be extensive and painful. Sometimes urination is so painful a woman has to be hospitalized for urinary retention. When the blisters break, craterlike lesions are revealed that can sometimes become infected with bacteria. Eventually, the lesions heal without scarring. The virus can then hide, or become dormant in nerves, until the next outbreak. Often stress, such as an illness, or the start of mens, will cause another episode.

391

Q Is it dangerous to have herpes while you are pregnant?

A Pregnant women who have herpes are monitored very carefully near the time of delivery because the disease is devastating to a newborn. Cultures may be done if the mother doesn't have any obvious lesions to make sure the disease isn't active. A pregnant woman with a history of herpes should notify her doctor immediately if she thinks she may be in labor or has leaking fluid.

392

Q Can a woman transmit herpes to her partner if she doesn't have any active lesions?

A Although women are most infectious during an active outbreak, and should avoid intercourse at that time, studies show they sometimes spread the virus when there are no active lesions. Taking suppressive medications may decrease the chance of viral shedding. A woman should share her history of herpes with potential sexual partners.

393

Q Is it dangerous to take medication for a long time to prevent herpes outbreaks?

A The herpes antiviral medications seem to be relatively safe and risk free even though there aren't any long-term studies that address continuous use.

394

Q How can a woman tell if a lesion on her vulva lips is herpes or something else?

A A physician can order a viral culture to diagnose the lesion. The newer the lesions, the more likely the culture will detect a virus if it is present.

395

Q How should a woman approach a prospective partner about the subject of herpes?

A When contemplating an intimate relationship with another person, it is important to tell them at once that you have had herpes in the past, when your last outbreak occurred, if there are any current lesions, and the medication being taken, if any. This type of conversation will encourage both people to be open and honest about their sexual histories.

396

Q Do people still get syphilis?

A Syphilis, an old STD disease that is usually treated with modern antibiotics such as penicillin, is actually on the rise. It is usually spread by sexual contact and produces a painless shallow ulcer called a chancre. The chancre will clear up untreated. Some people will get a rash over the whole body, inflammation of the covering of the brain, and damage to the heart, blood vessels, or spinal cord. In its late stages, syphilis can cause dementia, poor coordination, and stroke.

397

Q How is syphilis detected?

A Syphilis is a spirochete organism that cannot be cultured outside the body. Diagnosis is based on a blood screening test called a VDRL. If the test is abnormal, another specific test is done to check for the disease. Syphilis is not the only disease that could cause a positive VDRL.

398

Q Can syphilis cause any problems during pregnancy?

A Syphilis can cross the placenta and cause birth defects after the sixteenth week of pregnancy. All women at risk should be screened for syphilis early in their pregnancy and treated immediately if they are positive.

399

Q What are the risk factors for syphilis?

A Like all sexually transmitted diseases, the risk of syphilis is related to the number of sexual partners and the prevalence of unprotected intercourse. The transmission of the disease can occur even with the use of a condom if the lesion is not covered by the condom. People who are HIV positive have a higher risk of syphilis. It is important to treat all sexual partners to control the spread of the disease.

400

Q How is syphilis treated?

A Syphilis infections can be divided into several different stages, and the stage of syphilis a woman is in determines the treatment she receives. The early stage is usually easily cured by a single injection of penicillin. Tetracycline can be used as an alternative drug for people who are allergic to penicillin. Later stages of syphilis require other evaluations, such as a spinal tap, before treatment can be determined.

401

Q What is a trichomonas infection?

A Trichomonas vaginitis (trich) is the third most common form of vaginitis. It is an STD caused by a one-celled organism called a protozoan. Many men with the infection have no symptoms.

402

Q What are the symptoms for women of trichomonas?

A Although some women with trichomonas don't experience any symptoms, most have an itchy, discolored, foul-smelling vaginal discharge. Trichomonas can also cause an inflammation of the lining of the urethra (urethritis), producing pain with urination.

403

Q How is the diagnosis of trichomonas made?

A A physician or nurse usually tests for this type of infection after hearing the symptoms and seeing the vaginal tissue and discharge. A microscopic examination of the vaginal fluid will show the one-celled organism "swimming" in the vaginal fluid.

404

Q How is trichomonas treated?

A There is an antibiotic, called metronidazole, that is effective in treating trich infections. All sexual partners should be treated at the same time to avoid continual transmission of the STD.

405

Q What are scabies?

A Scabies are tiny mites that burrow under the skin and cause intense itching. They can be transmitted by sexual contact or by infected clothes, linens, or furniture. Over-the-counter medications are available to treat scabies.

Aches, Pains, and Fatigue

406

Q Why do women tend to experience more aches, pains, and stiffness as they get older?

A As the body ages, the joints start to literally wear out, and the ligaments, tendons, and muscles are not as flexible. Chronic diseases such as arthritis become more common. Some suggest the natural fall of the hormone DHEA as the body ages causes some of these symptoms. (DHEA is a weak male hormone produced in the adrenal glands and the ovaries; it sometimes referred to as a "pro" hormone because it can be metabolized into estrogen.) Exercising to keep strong and flexible can compensate for part of the natural aging process. Supplements such as DHEA are being tried by some to help slow the process.

407

Q What does arthritis mean?

A Arthritis means inflammation of the joint. There are many types of arthritis. All of the varieties have painful, tender, and sometimes red and swollen joints in common.

408

Q What is osteoarthritis?

A Osteoarthritis is a result of wearing out of the cartilage in a joint that is used as a cushion to prevent the ends of the bones from rubbing together. When the cartilage is worn out or gone, the bones rub together causing irritation, inflammation, pain, and sometimes bone spurs. Osteoarthritis is more common in the weight-bearing joints such as the knee, hip, and spine. It is treated by physical therapy and anti-inflammatory medications most often. Joint replacement may be suggested in some cases.

409

Q What is rheumatoid arthritis?

A This type of arthritis is an autoimmune disease with chronic, progressive inflammation of the lining of the joints. The afflicted joints are usually swollen, red, and tender to the touch. People of any age can have the disease. Much of the deformity of the joints can be avoided by early diagnosis and control of the inflammation with medications.

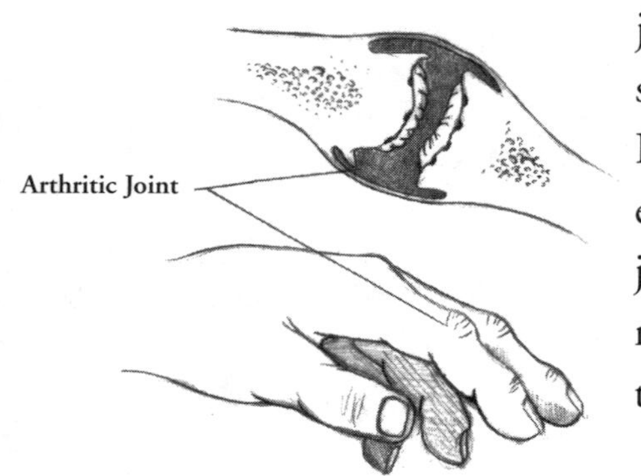

410

Q What can be done to alleviate knee pain when walking for exercise?

A It is important to have knees evaluated by a physician if there is swelling, redness, or pain. Treating the knees with ice packs after exercise will decrease pain. An over-the-counter anti-inflammatory pain reliever will often decrease soreness. Doing the same activity every day may overwork certain parts of the body. Other exercises should be performed, such as water aerobics, which take pressure off the knees.

411

Q How could a woman who doesn't play tennis get tennis elbow?

A Tennis elbow, or tendinitis, refers to the inflammation of a cord of tissue, a tendon, that connects muscles to the bone. Although repetitive use of the tendon in sports often causes tendinitis, the same type of repetitive use can occur from everyday activities such as using a screwdriver or painting.

412

Q How is tendinitis treated?

A Ice, rest, and anti-inflammatory drugs are used to treat the inflammation. Steroid injections are sometimes used for quick relief, but the problem can recur. Decreasing the repetitive activity is the first step towards healing. Physical therapy to improve muscle strength, or a brace to decrease the stress on certain tendons, may allow the return of activity with less pain.

413

Q Why does a woman sometimes wake up with lower back pain?

A The spine is a complex structure that supports our upright posture. There are jelly-filled disks between each of the twenty-four vertebra that cushion the spaces between the bones. Sometimes these disks can rupture (a slipped, or herniated, disk) and put pressure on the nearby nerve that comes out of the spinal

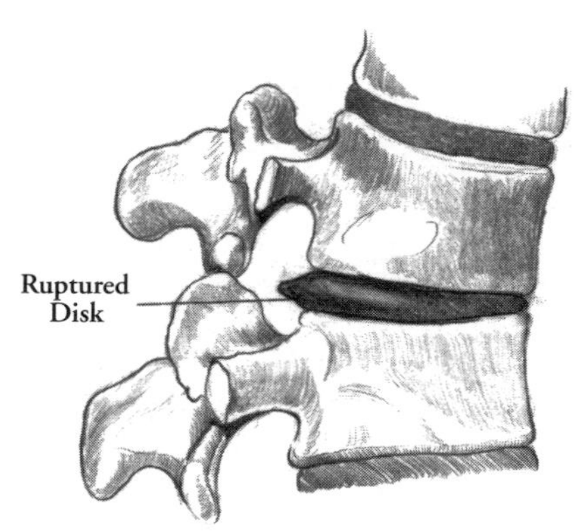

cord. Anything that puts pressure on these nerves can cause pain, numbness, or paralysis. Back pain can result from muscle spasms, vertebrae fractures as in osteoporosis, cancer that has spread to the bones, tumors, infection, or slipped disks. Sometimes kidney infections can also cause back pain. If your back pain isn't cured by conventional measures such as rest, ice or heat, and over-the-counter pain medication, see your physician.

414

Q What can be done to prevent lower back pain?

A Keeping back and abdomen muscles strong and flexible definitely decreases the chance of back problems. Daily stretching of the lower back by lying on the floor and pulling the knees one at a time to the chest helps keep the muscles flexible. Doing crunches with a good neck support and the knees bent with the feet flat on the floor strengthens the abdomen. Wearing shoes with a low heel, controlling weight, and sitting and standing with good posture all decrease the risk of back problems.

415

Q Is surgery necessary for a ruptured disk in the back?

A Physical therapy to improve muscle strength and flexibility, medications to decrease inflammation, and rest are the conservative therapies that are used. If this fails after several months, or if there are functional problems, such as weakness of a muscle group or numbness, surgery may be needed to remove the disk. Discuss your options with an orthopedic surgeon and consider getting a second opinion as well.

416

Q What might be wrong with a woman who has trouble getting out of bed in the morning and can't wait to get back in at night?

A Many diseases, including depression, cause excessive fatigue. The place to start an evaluation is with a good medical history and physical examination by a health-care provider. This should be followed by blood studies, including a biochemistry profile of over twenty different tests, a complete blood count, a TSH to rule out thyroid problems, and a urinalysis. Other tests may be recommended based on your individual circumstances.

417

Q What's the next step if there is no medical answer for exhaustion?

A No medical evaluation is perfect, and a second opinion may be warranted if symptoms persist. However, a woman should look at her life objectively for clues to exhaustion: unreasonable schedule of activities, lack of exercise, unhealthy eating, major life changes, or loss of a loved one.

418

Q Is chronic fatigue syndrome real?

A Chronic fatigue is a syndrome characterized by severe tiredness and a variety of other physical and mental complaints such as depression, joint pain, sleep disturbances, muscle pain, headaches, exercise intolerance, sore throat, enlarged painful lymph nodes, impaired memory, irritability, and difficulty concentrating. There may be a number of chronic fatigue syndromes with different causes. Although there is no real understanding of what causes the syndrome, one theory is that an infection with a bacteria or virus may be the initial event that starts the immune imbalance that leads to the chronic fatigue.

419

Q How is chronic fatigue diagnosed?

A There are no definitive laboratory tests so the diagnosis is made clinically by a physician. The Centers for Disease Control states that a diagnosis can be made if: the fatigue interferes with work or other activities; the fatigue has been present for at least six months; the patient has at least four other symptoms present for six months that are associated with the disease; and a physician can rule out any other causes of the fatigue.

420

Q How is chronic fatigue treated?

A The health-care provider recommends lifestyle changes and limitations on activities that make the woman feel worse. Using an antidepressant, education, and support groups to help patients and their families are all helpful in coping with the illness.

421

Q What is fibromyalgia?

A Fibromyalgia is a syndrome characterized by stiff, painful muscles, ligaments, and tendons. It is most common in middle-aged women who also have sleep disturbances and fatigue. The symptoms from this disorder may spontaneously regress to recur at a later time. There is a considerable overlap in symptoms with chronic fatigue and other muscle pain syndromes.

422

Q Is there any way to treat fibromyalgia?

A Physical therapy, stretching, massage, and aerobic exercise are all important. Tricyclic antidepressants at bedtime, such as Elavil, and muscle relaxants are often helpful. This is not a progressive, debilitating disease but may cause significant distress to patients and their families. Education and support groups are available in most areas.

423

Q How can a person who feels fine be anemic?

A Anemia is diagnosed when the number of red blood cells is low or the amount of hemoglobin in each cell is deficient. Mild anemia usually has no symptoms. Because red blood cells carry oxygen to the body's tissues, moderate anemia can cause fatigue and decreased ability to exercise. More severe forms can cause a sore mouth or tongue, faintness, difficulty swallowing, headaches, abnormal fingernails, weight loss, and other gastrointestinal symptoms.

424

Q What causes anemia?

A Although thalassemia and sickle-cell anemia are inherited forms of the disease, the most common cause is iron deficiency. Women lose more iron during their reproductive years than they absorb from their diet. A significant source of iron is lost when women eat less red meat to decrease their intake of cholesterol and saturated fat. Starvation, whether self-imposed or from living conditions, causes the body to use up its iron. In addition, vitamin deficiencies such as folic acid and the inability to absorb vitamin B-12 can cause anemia.

425

Q How is pernicious anemia treated?

A Pernicious anemia occurs when the stomach cannot absorb vitamin B-12. Injections of the vitamin are given to these women to prevent the disease. If not treated correctly, the deficiency can cause serious neurological disorders. Patients with pernicious anemia need to be under the care of a physician.

426

Q Is there anything a woman can do to prevent passing on thalassemia to her children?

A People who carry this trait, or sickle-cell anemia, should have genetic counseling prior to pregnancy. A counselor will review family histories, suggest testing for both partners, and present options for the management of the risk to any children.

427

Q What can be done about severe leg cramps that occur in the middle of the night?

A It sometimes helps to increase the flexibility of the leg muscles with gentle, consistent stretching exercises. A warm bath or heating pad decreases the incidence of cramps for some while others find help from ice packs. Still other women take a nonprescription dose of quinine, 200 to 300 mg before bedtime. Pregnant women or those with an enzyme deficiency such as G6PD shouldn't take quinine.

428

Q What is restless leg syndrome?

A People who suffer from restless leg syndrome have a strange sensation in their legs just before they start to fall asleep. The sensation like bugs crawling under their skin is so severe they can't keep their legs still. No one understands what causes it, and the problem often resolves itself after about an hour. Sedatives are helpful but can be habit forming. Exercise, stretching, and using hot or cold packs can also be beneficial.

429

Q What is heartburn?

A Gastroesophageal reflux disease is often called heartburn. Reflux of gastric acid can cause, in a severe case, ulceration and narrowing of the esophagus. Some foods, such as raw onions, spicy food, and alcohol, can aggravate the problem.

430

Q Is there anyway to treat heartburn?

A Raising the head of the bed four to six inches off the ground helps prevent reflux. Simply adding pillows doesn't work. Several new drugs are available to decrease the production of stomach acid and help the stomach speed up digestion of the food. In addition, several over-the-counter medications, such as Tagamet, are available.

431

Q What should a woman do to help her feet when they are killing her by the end of the day?

A Good foot care begins with keeping feet clean and dry and toenails carefully trimmed. Wearing shoes that fit is crucial. Lower heels and insoles will keep the feet comfortable.

Custom shoe inserts, orthodics, can be made from a mold of the woman's feet.

432

Q What is a bunion?

A A bunion is a boney protrusion that sticks out from the base of the big toe. Wearing poorly fitted, high-heeled shoes with narrow toes escalates this problem. As might be expected, women have three times as many bunions as men.

433

Q Is there anyway to avoid bunions?

A It's not clear, but the tendency to develop a bunion is probably genetic. Nevertheless, wearing properly fitted shoes with insoles, avoiding prolonged standing, and using an anti-inflammatory medication when necessary can often control the symptoms. In some cases, surgery may be recommended.

434

Q Why type of surgery is necessary to remove a bunion?

A A bunionectomy is usually done under local anesthesia as a day surgical procedure. Sometimes surgery is the only effective treatment to allow a woman to wear normal shoes and walk without pain. The six-month recovery has the woman wearing special shoes to protect the foot. In some cases, a cast is recommended.

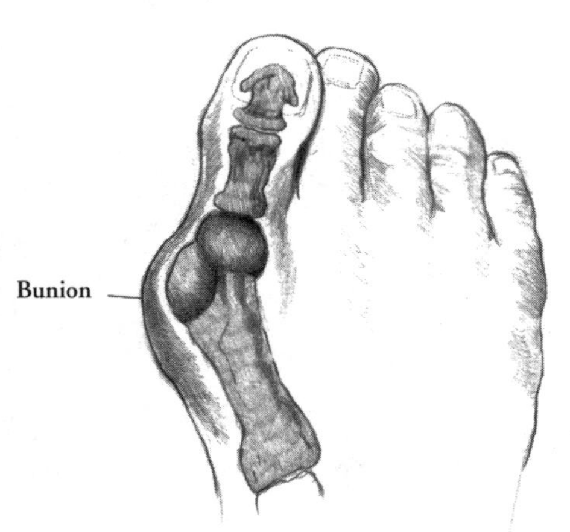

435

Q What type of problem does a woman have when her heel hurts first thing in the morning when she starts to walk on it?

A When a woman has been off her feet for awhile and exerts pressure to walk, pain may be caused by plantar fasciitis, an inflammation of the fibrous tissue. Similar problems can occur with bone spurs. Conservative therapy such as an anti-inflammatory drug, shoe inserts, taping the foot temporarily, and occasional steroid injections can improve the pain. It is important to be diagnosed by a physician, orthopedic surgeon, or podiatrist.

436

Q Can anything be done for an ingrown toenail?

A An ingrown toenail occurs when the edge of the nail curls under and digs into the soft tissue of the nail bed. Wearing shoes that fit improperly is the most common cause of ingrown toenails. Fungal infections and foot deformities can increase the risk or aggravate ingrown toenails. Signs of infection include swelling, redness, pus, and increased pain. Medical assistance is necessary at the first sign of infection. This is especially dangerous in diabetics, who should have regular medical foot care.

437

Q What causes a woman's knees to hurt when she goes down stairs or kneels down?

A Anterior knee pain is much more common in women than in men. Pain is usually felt right behind the knee cap and is exacerbated by certain activities. Usually the knee cap is pulled to one side by tight supporting ligaments. Physical therapy, regular exercise, or both can often improve this condition significantly. Ice packs, pain medication, and anti-inflammatory medications can suppress flare-ups. An orthopedic surgeon should be consulted for recurrent knee pain. A good physical examination and X rays will rule out arthritis or any other disease.

438

Q What is a torn cartilage in the knee?

A There are wedge-shaped pieces of cartilage in the knee that cushion the thigh and lower leg bones. If one of these is torn, whether from athletic activity or arthritis, the patient often experiences a painful clicking or popping sensation when the knee is bent or rotated. The knee may also seem to "give way" or lock.

439

Q How is a torn cartilage treated?

A A torn cartilage in the knee is treated conservatively with ice, rest, and anti-inflammatory medications such as Naprosyn or ibuprofen. Many people will improve or completely recover with this therapy followed by physical rehabilitation to strengthen the muscles around the knee. Others require a day surgery procedure called arthroscopy. An orthopedic surgeon can look into the joint and sometimes remove the torn pieces of cartilage looking through a fiber optic scope inserted into the knee joint. In this case, physical therapy is still necessary to rehabilitate the joint. The results depend on the success of the surgery and the patient's willingness to follow through with a physical therapy regimen.

440

Q What causes headaches?

A Three basic types of headaches are vascular (migraine), tension, and a combination of tension and vascular. Headaches can be caused by high blood pressure, a brain tumor, a sinus infection, temporal arteritis, temporomandibular joint (TMJ) syndrome, an infection of the central nervous system (meningitis), and hormonal changes that accompany a menstrual cycle, among other things.

441

Q How does a woman decide when to go to a doctor for a headache?

A There are several warning signs that indicate the need to seek medical attention for a headache: (1) A severe headache accompanied by fever and stiff neck; (2) a severe unrelenting headache unlike any you have ever experienced; (3) any headache that is accompanied by difficulty speaking, prolonged numbness, double vision, or imbalance; (4) a headache that begins in the temporal area, affects vision, and isn't relieved by simple pain relievers; (5) and a headache that persists even after treatment with pain medication.

442

Q How can a woman recognize if she is having a migraine headache?

A Migraine, or vascular, headaches often start on one side of the head with moderate to severe throbbing. The pain may be accompanied by nausea, vomiting, and aversion to light (photophobia). There is often localization of the pain behind one eye or in the temple region. Although the cause is unknown, some studies show vascular constriction is followed by dilation.

443

Q What is a headache aura?

A A migraine headache may be preceded by an aura thirty to sixty minutes prior to the onset of pain as a warning. Common auras are visual and include zigzag lines, colored lights, flashes of light, black holes, and blind spots. Less common warning signs are numbness or tingling in an extremity, hallucination, or speech changes.

444

Q Are there any triggers for a migraine?

A Aged cheese, red wine, smoked or cured meat, chocolate, coffee, tea, chicken livers, nitrates (preservatives used in hot dogs and other foods), and MSG (monosodium glutamate) found in many canned and Oriental foods tend to be triggers. Each woman needs to determine the specific foods that affect her.

445

Q Why do migraine headaches sometimes seem to be triggered by sinus problems?

A Sinus headaches can trigger migraines. Treatment of the sinus problem, allergies, or obstruction in the sinus area may significantly decrease the frequency of migraines.

446

Q How can a woman tell if she has a tension headache?

A Tension, or muscle contraction, headaches are common and feel like a band is tightening around the head. The pain may radiate down the back of the neck. Tension headaches may start in the morning, are more common in the afternoon, and get worse as the day progresses. Relaxation techniques and stress reduction exercises are helpful in decreasing the incidence and severity of these types of headaches.

447

Q Why would one woman's headaches get better on birth control pills and another's get worse?

A Some women report improvement in the frequency and severity of headaches on the pill while others don't. Birth control pills produce even hormone levels that are less likely to trigger migraines. Some women only get headaches the week they are off the active pills.

448

Q Why do some women have more sinus headaches when it gets humid?

A Many people have allergies to mold spores that grow quickly when it is wet and humid. Check the local mold spore count through the newspaper, television, or local American Lung Association. A dehumidifier that removes humidity from the air can be used in a home or office to lower the level of mold.

13

Eyes, Ears, Nose, and Throat

449

Q Why would a woman's ear hurt when her doctor says it looks normal?

A The jaw is connected to the skull by the temporomandibular joint (TMJ). It is common for people with a lot of stress, or misaligned teeth, to grind their teeth, which puts added stress on the joint. There may be a popping or clicking sound when the jaw is moved. Some forms of arthritis can also settle in this joint causing pain and deformity. The pain may originate in this joint but be felt in the ear. Tooth infections or other dental problems can also cause the person to feel pain coming from her ear.

450

Q How is TMJ syndrome evaluated?

A A physician or dentist reviews the symptoms and carefully evaluates the joint for pain, abnormal movement, and swelling. An X ray or MRI (magnetic resonance imaging) may be done to look for degeneration of the joint cartilage or bone spurs. A plastic mouth guard worn at night will decrease the grinding of the teeth as well as the ultimate wear of the joint. Over-the-counter pain relievers, muscle relaxants, and anti-inflammatory medications are helpful to alleviate discomfort. Braces to realign teeth and surgery may be required in some cases.

451

Q What causes the feeling that a room is spinning?

A Vertigo causes a woman to feel like the room is moving or spinning. This sensation is most often caused by a viral infection of the inner ear. The symptoms will resolve over time and are controlled by medication such as Antevert (meclizine). Because tumors and other disorders can sometime causes the same feeling, a physician should reevaluate the condition if the symptoms persist.

452

Q What would cause a woman to feel dizzy?

A There are many reasons a woman might feel dizzy. The momentary feeling of dizziness that sometimes comes from getting up too fast from a sitting or lying position is called postural hypotension. If this is a common problem for you, you should have your blood count and blood pressure checked by your doctor.

453

Q Is it normal for a woman to have trouble hearing as she gets older?

A Many people experience a gradual decrease in hearing acuity but can still hear adequately as they age. A physician should be contacted for any sudden decrease in hearing, which indicates a problem.

Part I ***Understanding Today's Health-Care System***

1 A Conversation with Nancy and Jane

Part II ***The Phases of Life***

2 Puberty

3 Menstruation

4 Pregnancy

5 Menopause

6 Osteoporosis

7 Aging Gracefully

Part III ***A Look at the Body***

8 The Female Breast

9 The Reproductive Organs

10 The Digestive Tract

11 Sexuality and Sexually Transmitted Diseases

12 Aches, Pains, and Fatigue

13 Eyes, Ears, Nose, and Throat

454

Q Why do some women have trouble hearing in noisy, crowded places?

A People with noise-induced hearing loss often have this type of complaint. If you are experiencing this, you should be tested by an audiologist. A hearing aid may help you overcome this type of hearing problem.

455

Q What causes a woman to hear ringing in her ears when it gets very quiet?

A Tinnitus is the sensation of ringing in the ears. The most common cause is noise-induced hearing loss. However, high blood pressure, excessive aspirin use, or rare tumors of the auditory nerve could be the cause. A physician should be contacted for an evaluation.

456

Q Why would eating Chinese food cause a woman's ears to ring?

A If a woman is overly sensitive to monosodium glutamate (MSG), which is commonly found in Chinese food, this can be a common symptom. Most restaurants will remove the MSG if asked.

457

Q What is Ménière's syndrome?

A The symptoms of Ménière's syndrome are vertigo, ringing in the ears, fluctuating hearing loss, and a sense of fullness or stuffiness in the ears. No one knows what causes this syndrome, but there are medications that can reduce some of these symptoms.

458

Q Why do some people snore so loudly?

A Snoring is a sign of blockage or obstruction of the airway. It is most often caused by floppy tissue in the back of the throat or enlarged tonsils. Being overweight or having allergies can contribute to the problem.

459

Q Is there anything that can be done for snoring?

A Some helpful hints are to sleep on the side rather than on the back; avoid antihistamines, sedatives, and alcohol near bedtime; and use an over-the-counter device called Breathe Right. A small pillow that fits under the back of the neck may help to decrease obstruction. Snoring can sometimes be dangerous. If you are concerned, seek a medical evaluation from a physician.

460

Q What is sleep apnea?

A Sleep apnea is a dangerous disorder. When an episode occurs, the sufferer will stop breathing during the course of sleep. Some experience a fall in the amount of oxygen in their blood, while others are at increased risk for heart arrhythmias and sudden death. A sleep study is the most comprehensive diagnostic tool to diagnosis true sleep apnea.

461

Q What are the treatments for sleep apnea?

A After a diagnosis is established, the patient can wear a positive-pressure breathing device, which fits into the nose or is given through a mask placed over the face at night. Another alternative is a surgical procedure that decreases the obstruction by removing excess tissue from the back of the throat. Weight loss will help some sufferers of sleep apnea.

462

Q What causes a woman's ears to feel like they are plugged up a lot of the time?

A Sometimes the external ear canal becomes blocked with too much wax. Ear cleaning kits are available from the drugstore for home use. A health-care provider should be contacted if the ears do not clear and hearing is affected. Don't use cotton swabs or other devices to clean out your ears. They can damage the tympanic membrane or ear canal.

463

Q Why would a woman's ears feel clogged up when the nurse says they are clear of wax buildup?

A The Eustachian tube runs from the middle ear to the back of the nose. Pressure builds up in the ears when this small tube becomes blocked or swollen shut, causing the ears to feel clogged. Allergies and colds are the most common causes of this type of problem. A physician should be consulted if the woman experiences this problem on a regular basis.

464

Q What causes a woman's ears to hurt and make them feel like they are popping on an airplane?

A The eardrum is stretched, causing pain, when the pressure in the airplane cabin does not equal the pressure in a woman's ears. Swallowing, chewing gum, or sucking on a candy helps to open the Eustachian tube to equalize the ear pressure and alleviate the pain.

465

Q Are there over-the-counter medications available to help a woman's ears when she has to fly with allergies or a cold?

A Taking a decongestant, with an antihistamine, such as Tavist D, Dimetapp, Triaminic, or Sudafed Plus, may help decrease the swelling and allow the Eustachian tube to stay open. Using an Afrin-type nasal spray treatment before boarding the plane will open nasal and ear passages. Continual use of nasal sprays can be habit forming and will cause a rebound effect of symptoms so be sure to use it only when necessary.

466

Q What should a woman do if over-the-counter medications don't help her blocked ears?

A A physician can prescribe antihistamines or decongestants that are not available over the counter. Even though these types of medications help to shrink nasal membranes and open the Eustachian tube, they can increase heart rate and blood pressure and cause trouble sleeping. A minimally sedating antihistamine like Claritin, Allegra, or Zyrtec can be given alone or with a decongestant. Claritin D contains both an antihistamine and decongestant.

467

Q Does a woman need to be taking antihistamines regularly to control allergies?

A There are steroid nasal sprays that can be used daily to decrease allergic reactions in the nose and sinuses with minimal side effects. The medication acts on the tissues in the nose to decrease swelling and irritation. Some patients will need an antihistamine-decongestant and a steroid nasal spray to control symptoms. It's also recommended that a physician be seen for an evaluation because allergy testing and desensitization may be necessary.

468

Q How does the doctor test for allergies?

A There are two ways to test for allergies. One method is to place a tiny amount of the substance to be tested under the skin with a needle to determine a reaction. The newest method is to measure the body's antibody response to pollens, molds, dust, and pets through a blood test. The doctor can evaluate the results of either method to see if allergy shots or other treatment may be warranted.

469

Q Why do some women get a sinus infection every time they get a cold or their allergies act up?

A The swelling and mucus from a viral infection (cold) or allergies blocks the openings to the sinuses. Bacteria starts to grow when the sinuses don't drain, and the result is an infection. Infections can often be avoided if medications are taken to keep the sinuses draining.

470

Q What should a woman do if the sinus medications don't seem to work?

A A physician or an ear, nose, and throat specialist (ENT) should be consulted for a complete evaluation. Special X rays or scans can be taken of the sinuses to determine if there are any blockages, such as polyps, that need to be removed.

471

Q Is something wrong if a woman can't breathe through one side of her nose?

A The nasal septum is the structure that divides the nose into two halves. It may be bent, blocking one or sometimes both sides of the nose. Often an ENT specialist can surgically straighten the septum to improve breathing.

472

Q Why do some women's noses get stuffed up when they are around cigarette smoke?

A Smoke from tobacco products, like other environmental pollutants, can trigger an allergic reaction in nasal tissues. This causes the release of histamine, which causes swelling, increased mucus, and itching.

473

Q What can be done to decrease allergic symptoms?

A Antihistamines should be taken if avoidance of an allergen is not possible. Steroid nasal sprays that are taken regularly will decrease the reaction of the tissues to allergens, and avoiding secondhand smoke is very important.

474

Q What causes sinus headaches?

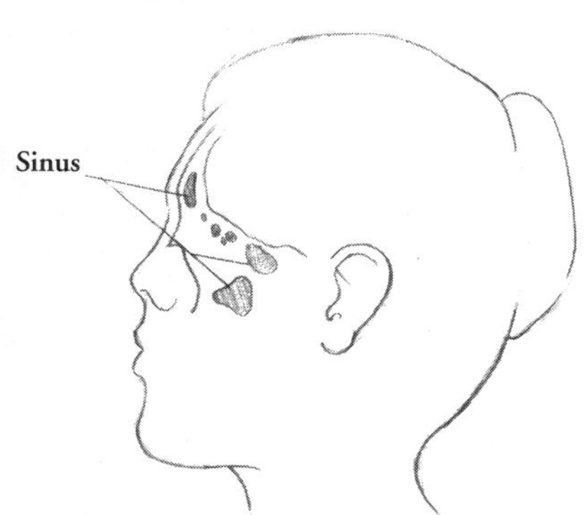

A Sinus headaches are most often caused by swelling of the nasal tissues, which is usually brought on by allergies. When the opening to the sinuses are blocked with mucus, pressure builds up and causes the pain. The pain will increase if an infection develops. Treating allergies to allow the sinuses to drain and using antibiotics to control the infection often relieve the symptoms. Endoscopic sinus surgery may be necessary if other treatments don't work.

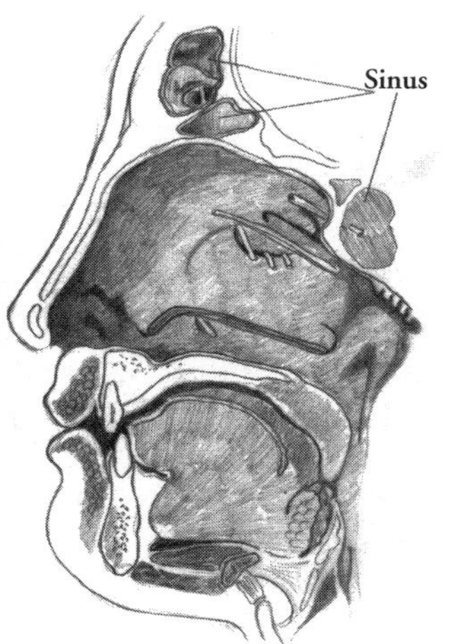

475

Q What are cataracts?

A Cataracts appear as clouding of the lens, which focuses light into the eye. This is a gradual process that escalates to impair vision. Although cataracts can happen at any age, they are more common in people over sixty years old. Diabetics are at risk for cataracts if their blood sugar levels are not controlled.

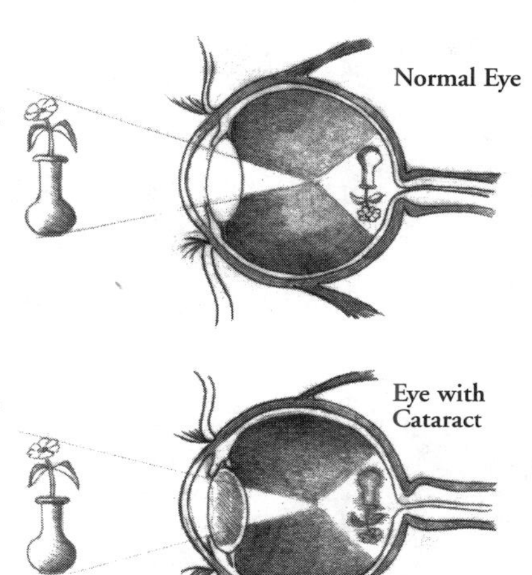

476

Q Can cataracts be prevented?

A Very little is known about cataracts except it is a chemical change in the lens substance that is related to aging. Wearing sunglasses to block ultraviolet light may be helpful. Although there are no good scientific studies, vitamins C and E and other antioxidants may be beneficial.

477

Q How are cataracts treated?

A The only successful treatment for cataracts is to remove the diseased lens and replace it with an artificial one. The woman will continue to need reading glasses after the procedure. As with all surgeries, there is always risk, but this procedure is generally safe and effective.

478

Q What has caused my eyes to be so dry?

A Dry eyes are very common and associated with aging. Menopause seems to trigger the problem in some women. Dry eyes, mouth, and lips are common symptoms of a connective tissue disorder called Sjogren syndrome. You should visit your doctor regularly to check your eyes for disease and vision changes. If you have a recurring problem with dryness, he can recommend a good moisturizing drop.

479

Q What is glaucoma?

A Glaucoma is characterized by an increase in the pressure of the fluid in the eye. This increased pressure damages the optic nerve at the back of the eye, leading to loss of vision. Fluid is constantly produced and drained out of the eye. The production and drainage are in balance to maintain a constant pressure. If more fluid is produced than is drained or re-absorbed, the pressure increases. Severe glaucoma will cause blindness.

480

Q Who is likely to get glaucoma?

A About 15 percent of people over eighty years old have chronic glaucoma. It becomes more common in increasing years. It is also more likely to affect African-Americans, diabetics, and those with a family history.

481

Q What do nearsighted and farsighted mean?

A If a woman is nearsighted she sees objects clearly if they are near while those at a distance appear blurry. The reverse is true for a woman who is farsighted. She sees objects clearly at a distance but not close-up. These eye problems are caused by abnormalities in the shape of the eyeball. As the eye ages, the lenses loose elasticity and do not change shape quickly enough to give clear close and distance vision. Women tend to become more farsighted as they age.

482

Q Is surgery to improve vision without glasses safe?

A A microsurgical procedure called radial keratotomy can permanently improve vision. It is primarily used to correct nearsightedness. Nine out of ten people who have this surgery are able to drive a car without glasses; some have excellent vision. If the procedure is not successful, the alteration in the shape of the cornea may prevent future use of contact lenses. Keratotomy is not always successful and about one in a thousand procedures can result in loss of vision due to infection.

483

Q What is astigmatism?

A Astigmatism is a condition caused by an irregularly shaped cornea, which is the transparent covering on the outside of the eye. This condition causes blurred vision and can be corrected by special types of contact lenses or corrective glasses.

484

Q What's the difference between an ophthalmologist and an optometrist?

A An ophthalmologist is a medical doctor who specializes in diseases of the eye. This type of physician can treat eye disorders with medication and surgery in addition to prescribing lenses. An optometrist is specially trained in evaluation of the eye and can prescribe glasses and contact lenses. An optometrist will refer a patient to an ophthalmologist if a medical problem is found during an exam. A woman should consider seeing an ophthalmologist if diabetes, high blood pressure, elevated cholesterol, or a history of eye problems exists.

485

Q Why is a retinal detachment an emergency?

A The retina of the eye contains the cells that detect light and transmit signals to the optic nerve. A retinal detachment occurs when the retina peels away from the back of the eye. This is more common in nearsighted Caucasians and tends to runs in families. There may be a permanent loss of vision if it is not treated immediately.

486

Q What are the symptoms of a retinal detachment?

A A retinal detachment is usually painless. The patient may see as if a curtain is moving over part of their vision, flashing bright lights or sparks. Blurry vision that suddenly occurs and a marked increase in the number of "floaters," the small specks that seem to float across your vision as you move your eye, are signs of a possible retinal detachment. Contact an ophthalmologist immediately or go to the emergency room of a hospital if the symptoms persist.

487

Q How is retinal detachment treated?

A There are several different ways to treat a retinal detachment. Laser welding or cryotherapy may help a partial detachment. At times a complete retinal detachment can be treated with microsurgery. It is extremely important to get immediate medical care because a significant delay reduces the chance of restoring sight.

488

Q What is macular degeneration?

A This eye disease is the major cause of blindness in the United States and other Western countries. The macula processes information about light from the retina and sends it to the brain. Degeneration of this part of the eye causes central vision to fade. The patient experiences trouble with tasks such as reading and driving a car but has enough vision to walk and perform daily tasks.

489

Q How is macular degeneration treated?

A Most forms of macular degeneration cannot be treated. The patient is taught to deal with the disability by using special reading glasses, large-print materials, and good lighting. Some studies show that increased use of green leafy vegetables (such as spinach, chard, and collard greens) may be able to decrease the risk of macular degeneration. Some physicians are beginning to prescribe antioxidant vitamins for this condition. Ocuvite is an over-the-counter vitamin rich in antioxidant vitamins, including zinc and selenium. This formulation, which targets free radicals, is aimed at slowing the progression of the disease.

490

Q Does my diet change or help protect my eyesight?

A There are several medical studies to suggest that eating foods rich in beta carotenoids (carrots, yellow squash, sweet potatoes, and pumpkins) may be helpful to eyesight. It is also a good idea to avoid excessive exposure to ultraviolet light.

491

Q What causes me to be hoarse and have to clear my throat?

A There are many benign causes of hoarseness such as straining the voice, post-nasal drainage from allergies, reflux of acid from the stomach, and benign vocal nodules. However, serious disease can be masked by the symptom. An evaluation by a physician will determine the severity of the problem.

492

Q How long should a woman wait to see a doctor if she is hoarse?

A Often a viral infection of the voice box, or larynx, can cause hoarseness that might last for a week or two. A doctor should be seen if the condition continues for more than two weeks.

493

Q Could a woman's throat be hoarse from singing on a regular basis?

A Straining the voice consistently, through singing or public speaking, will cause the formation of benign nodules on the vocal cords. Surgically removing the nodules will allow the physician to check for disease but will not correct the problem. The throat should be rested from excesses on a regular basis.

494

Q Can a woman continue to sing if she has vocal nodules?

A It's harmful to use the voice in excess when nodules are present. A speech therapist can teach a person to sing or talk for long periods of time without straining the voice.

Specific Medical Conditions

495

Q What is an aneurysm?

A An aneurysm is a weakness in the wall of a blood vessel that causes it to "balloon out" and eventually rupture. The aorta is the main blood vessel from the heart that distributes blood to most of the body. An aneurysm can occur in the aorta or other arteries such as the vessels in the brains. Rupture of an aneurysm is a medical emergency and can be fatal. An aneurysm is usually due to hardening of the arteries (atherosclerosis) and is more likely in older women with uncontrolled high blood pressure.

496

Q What is a pancreatitis attack?

A The pancreas is a glandular organ in the upper abdomen just behind the stomach. It has special cells that produce insulin. In addition, the pancreas produces enzymes that help digest food. The pancreas can become inflamed as a complication of gallbladder disease, a viral infection, alcohol intake, or exposure to certain drugs. This inflammation may be sudden and very painful (acute) or be recurrent (chronic). This is a potentially life-threatening disease that needs to be aggressively treated.

497

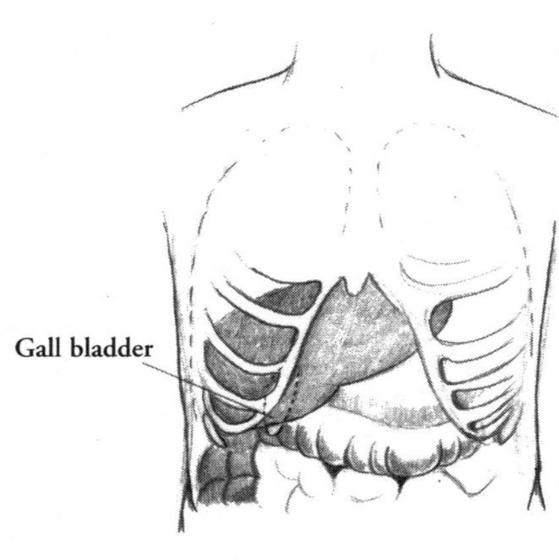

Q Why do women have more problems with gallstones than men?

A The gallbladder is a hollow organ on the underneath side of the liver. Women have twice as many gallbladder problems as men because the female hormones increase the rate of excretion of cholesterol stones into the gallbladder.

498

Q What are the symptoms of gallbladder problems?

A Most women with stones or an inflammation of the gallbladder notice pain or discomfort in the right upper part of the abdomen, especially after eating fatty foods. The pain may be felt more in the right shoulder or radiating through into the back rather than the abdomen. The pain may last for minutes or hours. An ultrasound study of the gallbladder can safely tell if gallstones are present.

499

Q What are a woman's options if she is diagnosed with gallstones?

A Some women have gallstones that never cause problems. However, complications from gallstones can be serious. Surgeons usually recommend that a diseased gallbladder be removed. Although most women are candidates for surgery through the laparoscope as an outpatient procedure using a general anesthetic, some will require a full incision with a hospital stay.

500

Q What is lupus?

A Lupus is a chronic autoimmune disorder that causes inflammation of collagen or connective tissue. The word lupus comes from the Latin word for "wolf" and refers to the rash that frequently appears on the face over the nose and cheeks. There are several different kinds of lupus, but generally the term refers to systemic lupus erythematosus, which afflicts ten times as many women as men.

501

Q What are the symptoms of lupus?

A Lupus can affect any area of the body. Initially, symptoms may be mild and come and go. A skin rash, sun sensitivity, arthritis, fatigue, hair loss, low-grade fever, and abdominal or chest pain can all be signs of the disease. The most severe symptoms are associated with damage to the kidney and heart or inflammation of the central nervous system causing problems with memory or even seizures. Some women have a mild form of the disease while others have a severe progressive disorder that is life threatening. African-American and Native American women tend to have the more severe form of the disease.

502

Q How is lupus diagnosed?

A People with lupus produce a variety of autoimmune antibodies. When the physician suspects lupus, a blood screening test called an antinuclear antibody (ANA) will be ordered. If it is positive, more definitive studies will be run to determine the exact diagnosis.

503

Q How is lupus treated?

A One of the drugs used to treat malaria, plaquenil, is often used to treat lupus. It decreases inflammation and has few side effects. Although steroids can have major side effects, they are sometimes used to suppress the production of autoimmune antibodies. Anti-inflammatory medications such as aspirin, ibuprofen, and Naprosyn are also effective in treating the arthritis symptoms of lupus. Women with the disease need to avoid sun exposure, which will worsen their rash.

504

Q What is scleroderma?

A Scleroderma is an autoimmune disorder where the skin becomes thickened, hard, and shiny. In some cases there are only mild skin changes. In other cases, where there is severe disease, there can be problems such as high blood pressure and damage to internal organs that causes difficulty swallowing and breathing. There is no cure but the symptoms can be treated with steroids.

505

Q What is Lyme disease?

A Lyme disease is an infection with a microorganism called a spirochete, which is spread to humans by infected ticks. There is sometimes a rash around the tick bite in a circle. Other symptoms include fatigue and joint pain. A blood test can be used to help determine if a person has Lyme disease. Antibiotics are most effective if the disease is found early.

506

Q What is multiple sclerosis?

A Multiple sclerosis (MS) is a chronic disease that attacks the central nervous system (the brain and spinal cord). Because random portions of nerve insulation are impaired, signals to parts of the body are slowed or blocked. Coordination, balance, vision, bowel or bladder function, and sexual function can all be altered by the disease. Some forms of the disease become increasingly worse over time while other forms are much milder and can include periods of complete remission. No cause has been found for MS.

507

Q What are the symptoms of multiple sclerosis?

A There are a variety of MS symptoms, including blurry vision, eye pain, difficulty walking, poor coordination, inability to control bowel or bladder function, numbness, and slurred speech. MS is difficult to diagnose because the symptoms are so diverse.

508

Q Who is most likely to get multiple sclerosis?

A MS is most often diagnosed in young people between the ages of twenty and forty. It is more common in people who grew up in the North than in the South and is neither inherited nor contagious. It does have a tendency to run in some families.

509

Q How is multiple sclerosis diagnosed?

A Diagnosis can be confusing because the symptoms of MS are so diverse. MS may be an autoimmune disorder although some researchers think it is a viral infection. Magnetic resonance imaging (MRI), as well as spinal taps, are helpful in diagnosis. The physician must look at the symptoms of the patient and laboratory evaluations to make this diagnosis.

510

Q How is multiple sclerosis treated?

A Corticosteroid drugs such as prednisone are helpful in diminishing severe attacks, but lifestyle changes that optimize diet, activity, and rest are crucial to disease management. Some cancer chemotherapy drugs, such as cytoxan and Imuran, are helpful but have many side effects. There is no known cure for multiple sclerosis and much more research is necessary to find a cause and develop an optimum treatment program.

511

Q What is carpal tunnel syndrome?

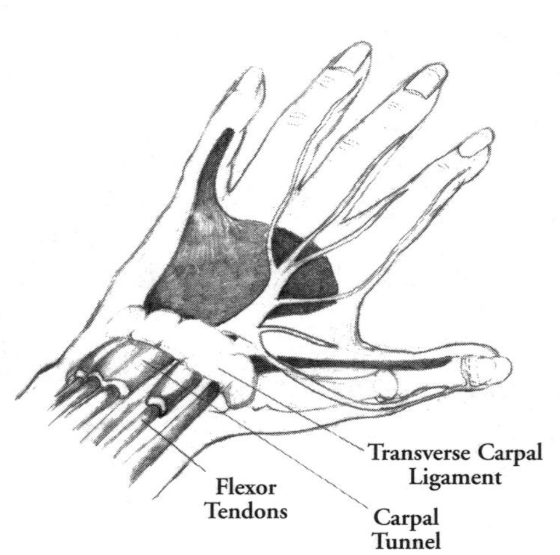

A Carpal tunnel syndrome is a painful syndrome that affects the wrists and hands. This affliction occurs most often in people who perform repetitive wrist movements such as typists, computer operators, gardeners, checkout clerks, and carpenters. The problem is caused by pressure on the median nerve, which moves through a narrow passageway called the carpal tunnel. This nerve connects to the thumb, index finger, middle finger, and inner part of the ring finger.

512

Q What are the symptoms of carpal tunnel syndrome?

A Initially the fingers involved with the median nerve feel numb or may tingle. The sensation escalates to pain, a burning sensation, and eventually numbness in the palm of the hand. Sometimes sharp, shooting pains can travel from the wrist to the palm and up into the forearm. Uncontrolled carpal tunnel can cause fingers to become permanently numb. In this case, muscles will deteriorate causing a severe disability.

513

Q How is carpal tunnel treated?

A Carpal tunnel problems have increased with the use of computer keyboards. Wearing splints to rest the wrist joint helps to decrease some pain and inflammation. Medications such as anti-inflammatory drugs or steroid injections are sometimes prescribed. In extreme cases, people have surgery to release the constriction of the carpal tunnel. A hand surgeon can make an incision over the ligament that binds the nerve under a local anesthetic. For many people, hand function returns and pain resolves within several months.

514

Q What is Raynaud's phenomenon?

A In this condition, fingers or toes, when cold or stressed, turn white then blue and finally red before they go back to normal. This disorder is more common in women than men and is sometimes associated with a connective tissue disorder such as scleroderma. Certain blood pressure medications, anticancer drugs, and nicotine increase the incidence of occurrence. Attacks can last from a few minutes to several hours.

515

Q How can Raynaud's be prevented?

A Avoiding the cold is a crucial preventative treatment for this condition. Gloves or mittens should be worn on hands that will be exposed to cold temperatures. A woman with Raynaud's should not smoke and should avoid smoky places. If you have other symptoms consistent with a connective tissue disorder, you should be evaluated by a rheumatologist.

516

Q What causes scoliosis?

A There is no known cause for scoliosis, which is a lateral "S" curvature of the spine. Children between the ages of ten and sixteen are routinely screened to find this problem early. Although many people experience a mild curvature without problems, others bear the physical disability of one shoulder blade protruding more than the other, uneven hips, a tilted waist, and a significant difference in lengths of their legs.

517

Q How is scoliosis treated?

A Many people with mild scoliosis don't require any treatment. A child who may be developing scoliosis should be evaluated by a physician who specializes in the disorder. Bracing is important for some patients and may prevent progression of the disease. Surgery may be necessary to stabilize the spine and correct deformity in patients with severe forms of scoliosis.

518

Q What is Turner's syndrome?

A Turner's syndrome is a genetic abnormality usually due to the absence of one X chromosome. Normal females have two X chromosomes (XX). Patients with Turner's syndrome have only one X chromosome; they are XO. Women with Turner's syndrome have a uterus but often no eggs in their ovaries. Although they have normal intelligence, these women tend to be short in height with a webbed deformity to the neck.

519

Q Why don't women with Turner's go through normal puberty or have periods?

A Because these women frequently don't produce eggs in their ovaries, they don't have estrogen to stimulate breast development or menstrual cycles. A physician uses medication, such as estrogen and progesterone, to cause normal sexual development and cycles. A woman with Turner's can choose to become pregnant by in vitro fertilization and egg donation.

520

Q What are shingles?

A This disease is the result of reactivating the virus that causes chicken pox (herpes zoster). This virus can live in nerves for many years and then be activated by stress, an immune deficiency, or poor health. It is more common in people over fifty years old. Almost 20 percent of people will have shingles at some time during their life.

521

Q What are the symptoms of shingles?

A The symptoms usually follow the path of a nerve root and begin with tingling and may progress to excruciating pain. Several days after the initial symptoms, blisters appear along the path of the affected nerve. The blisters will crust and usually resolve in three to four weeks. The pain and lesions may be gone in one to two weeks, or it may continue for months or years causing a chronic pain syndrome in some people. Although shingles are caused by the same virus as chicken pox, shingles are much less contagious. If shingles occur in the nerves to the eye, partial or total blindness can occur unless they are treated quickly.

522

Q How are shingles treated?

A Local symptoms of mild shingles can sometimes be treated with wet, cool compresses or lotions. However, many physicians recommend therapy with a medication called acyclovir. This oral medication, if started early and given in a dose of 800 mg five times daily for seven to ten days, will usually manage the pain of shingles and may help prevent long-term pain. In patients whose immune systems are compromised, such as people with AIDS or those undergoing chemotherapy, much higher doses of acyclovir may be necessary. Steroids like prednisone can also be used, but they have significant side effects. In the most severe cases of shingles, a combination of acyclovir and steroids may be necessary. Studies are currently underway for new antiviral drugs that may help shingles.

523

Q What is toxoplasmosis?

A This is an infection caused by a parasite found in undercooked meat and cat feces. Many people have the infection without any symptoms. If a pregnant woman acquires the disease during pregnancy, her fetus may become infected by placental transmission. Toxoplasmosis can cause miscarriage or birth defects ranging from eye problems to neurological disorders.

524

Q How can toxoplasmosis be prevented?

A Pre-pregnancy screening would be ideal to determine whether the woman has had the infection or is at risk for it. Once a woman has developed the antibodies for toxoplasmosis, she is no longer at risk for acquiring it. Pregnant women who have not developed the antibodies should avoid changing cat litter boxes or holding a cat near her face. If avoiding exposure is not possible, the woman should use gloves to change the litter box.

525

Q Can a woman who doesn't smoke get lung cancer?

A Most cases of lung cancer are the result of tobacco use. There also seems to be an increase in lung cancer that may be related to exposure to secondhand smoke and air pollution. However, some forms of lung cancer are not related to smoking. Women who have a chronic cough, cough up blood, or have chest pain or difficulty breathing should have a medical evaluation whether they smoke or not.

526

Q What is mono?

A Mononucleosis, "the kissing disease," is an infectious disease caused by the Epstein-Barr virus. It is generally spread by direct contact with body fluids. Many young people have the virus without symptoms. When symptoms flair to active disease, the person may feel extreme fatigue and weakness, have a sore throat, and have swollen lymph glands.

527

Q How is mononucleosis diagnosed?

A An initial screening blood test called a monospot can be ordered. If the monospot is positive, the diagnosis is made. If the woman has a negative monospot but symptoms consistent with mononeucleosis, a more specific test, Epstein-Barr virus titer, is performed. Liver enzyme tests are done in severe cases to determine if hepatitis is present. A complete blood count will often show atypical lymphocytes (a type of white blood cell) consistent with a viral infection.

528

Q Are there complications of mono?

A The virus can affect the liver and cause a form of hepatitis. In addition, because it may enlarge the spleen, rupture is possible and life threatening. People experiencing spleen enlargement should avoid contact sports or other high-risk activities. Any sharp sudden pain in the left upper part of the abdomen should be reported to a physician immediately.

529

Q What's the recovery time for mononucleosis?

A Most people are significantly improved in two to three weeks but experience the fatigue for an additional three or more months.

530

Q How is mono treated?

A There are no prescribed medications because mono is viral. Symptoms can be treated, however, with bedrest, plenty of water, and good nutrition. Nasal congestion is treated with decongestants while clinical examination or ultrasound is used to check the spleen. In severe cases, steroids such as prednisone can help decrease the sore throat and swollen lymph glands.

531

Q What is a cold?

A A cold is the common name for a viral infection of the upper respiratory tract. There are over two hundred viruses that can cause colds, making it unlikely that an effective vaccine will ever be developed. Most adults have three colds a year but young children can have six to ten. Healthy people will recover from a cold whether they seek medical attention or not. Colds account for the largest number of doctor visits each year.

532

Q How do you really catch a cold?

A Cold viruses can live on human skin for up to four hours and are spread by direct physical contact such as handshaking or sharing a telephone. The flu viruses are more likely to be spread through the air. Viral infections are more common in the winter because people spend more time crowded indoors.

533

Q What are the symptoms of a cold?

A The classic cold symptoms are runny, stuffy nose, sore throat, cough, and sometimes hoarseness. If there is a fever, it's rarely over one hundred degrees. Colds usually last a week or two.

534

Q When should a woman see a doctor for a cold?

A Although most colds are benign and last only a short time, there is the possibility of complications. The problem may start with a cold, which blocks the sinuses and can lead to a bacterial sinus infection that requires antibiotics. People with colds can develop middle ear infections that need to be treated. Contact a physician if a cold lasts more than three weeks or an earache, facial pain, greenish nasal discharge, persistent cough, wheezing, or high fever are present.

535

Q Do antibiotics help cure a cold?

A Antibiotics will do absolutely nothing for a cold. A cold is a viral illness that must run its course. Antibiotics will help, however, if there are complications from a cold such as a sinus or middle ear infection.

536

Q What is strep throat?

A Most sore throats are viral and, therefore, not responsive to antibiotics. Strep throat, however, is caused by a streptococcal bacteria that should be treated with an antibiotic. Only a throat culture will determine if the problem is truly the result of a strep infection. It is best to get a culture rather than going straight to therapy with an antibiotic you probably don't need.

537

Q What is insomnia?

A Insomnia can mean trouble getting to sleep (taking more than forty-five minutes), waking up frequently unable to fall back to sleep, or early morning awakening. Short-term insomnia, lasting from a few nights to a few weeks, is usually caused by worry over a stressful situation. Long-term insomnia, which can last months or even years, is often caused by general anxiety, medications, chronic pain, depression, or other physical disorders.

538

Q What symptoms does sleep deprivation cause?

A People who are chronically sleep deprived show signs of poor coordination, daytime sleepiness, poor concentration, poor judgment, and irritability. They often fall asleep when they don't plan to and are at risk for automobile accidents.

539

Q What causes people not to sleep well?

A Stress and depression can cause sleep problems. Any disease that makes sleep uncomfortable, such as fibromyalgia, arthritis, restless leg syndrome, or sleep apnea, can inhibit sleep. Taking caffeine, drugs that contain phentermine, phenylpropanolamine, or other stimulants is also known to keep people awake. Having to urinate after drinking excessive fluid late in the day as well as hot flushes from menopause also disturb sleep.

540

Q How can I prevent insomnia?

A Lifestyle and behavioral changes can be made to encourage good, restful sleep. Having regular sleep hours without a nap is key. Stressful activities or thought-provoking topics should be avoided close to bedtime. A calm sleep environment, with little noise, is ideal. Sometimes a bedtime ritual lets your mind and body know it is time for sleep. For example, an hour before bedtime you might take a warm bath, drink a cup of herbal, decaffinated tea, and then read for a few minutes before turning in.

541

Q Why do some people get thick ugly scars when they have a cut?

A Thick scars are called keloids and are due to an over-growth of scar tissue. Some women are susceptible to this type of scarring. Women from dark-skin ethnic groups more commonly have keloids than lighter skinned people.

542

Q Can keloids be prevented or treated?

A Treatment of keloids is difficult and not always successful. Injection of anti-inflammatory steroids into the scar may help decrease it. Surgical resection of the scar only makes another scar. Laser therapies may offer improved treatments in the future.

543

Q What is sick building syndrome (SBS)?

A Older, well-ventilated buildings have been increasingly replaced by newer, more efficient, airtight buildings since the 1970s, and there has been a corresponding increase in the reported incidence of sick building syndrome (SBS) since that time. The symptoms of patients with this problem are nonspecific and are not related to an infection or hypersensitivity syndrome. The symptoms tend to cluster among employees who work in the same building and are sometimes even localized to one floor or work area. Common symptoms include headache, upper respiratory irritation, fatigue, rash, itching, inability to concentrate, cough, and shortness of breath. Patients often report smelling unusual odors. The severity of the problem can vary greatly among the people exposed, and the people exposed can experience different symptoms. Typically, the symptoms appear when the people are exposed to the building environment and regress after they leave.

544

Q What causes SBS?

A Many factors can be responsible for sick building syndrome. Often there is not just one cause. New or newly remodeled buildings are at a greater risk for SBS. However, older buildings with dirty carpets and poor ventilation can also be affected. There are several theories on the cause of SBS, but inadequate ventilation and air contamination seem to be important risk factors.

545

Q How would a woman know if she was being exposed to SBS?

A A diagnosis is based on the occurrence of symptoms while employees are in the building and their consistent improvement away from the building. There should be symptoms in coworkers that cannot be attributed to other causes. If employees suspect SBS, they should request their employer to hire a consultant such as an industrial hygienist to initiate an investigation and perform an indoor air quality evaluation. If your building does have SBS, treatment of the building by improving ventilation or removing toxic substances or both will increase employee efficiency and decrease loss of work time.

546

Q What is multiple chemical sensitivity?

A Multiple chemical sensitivity (MCS) is a chronic condition in which the patient reacts to many different environmental, food, and chemical stimulants at levels well tolerated by most people. Patient reactions, for example, may include facial or chest pain, dizziness, chest tightness, shortness of breath, muscle spasms, nausea, headache, arthritis, swelling, watery eyes, and memory loss among other things. Some common triggering factors are exhaust fumes, cigarette smoke, solvents, perfumes, pesticides, disinfectants, grasses, molds, newsprint, and fabrics.

547

Q What causes MCS?

A Traditional medicinal investigations don't find any specific cause for these sensitivities. Patients with these complaints are often under the age of forty-five, female, and can be severely debilitated by their condition. Some "environmental ecologists" hypothesize that these people have an immune system that has been overwhelmed by environmental contaminants. They offer injections to desensitize patients to substances that provoke the response and teach avoidance techniques. These treatments are highly controversial and generally not supported by the traditional medical community. Others have suggested that MCS is really a conditioned response to a stimulus and may be successfully treated by classical desensitization techniques such as those used for agoraphobia (fear of unfamiliar surroundings).

548

Q What is epilepsy?

A Epilepsy is a term referring to a group of seizure disorders. A seizure is the result of excessive electrical activity in the brain that leads to abnormal movements, behaviors, or sensations. A seizure can be localized or involve the whole body. The most common seizure is the grand mal that affects the whole body. This is characterized by convulsive movements of the entire body and often loss of bladder or bowel control. Smaller seizures, referred to as petite mal, cause a momentary lapse of consciousness.

549

Q How are seizures treated?

A Most seizures can be controlled with medication. Dilantin and phenobarbital are two of the most common seizure medications. Avoidance of excessive use of alcohol, fatigue, exhaustion, and stress may decrease the incidence. Some people can find and avoid a specific trigger that most often initiates a seizure.

550

Q Do people with seizures have mental illnesses?

A Seizures are a medical illness and have nothing to do with intelligence or mental illness. A person with the disorder, however, may need counseling to help accept limitations they may encounter because of the seizure disorder.

551

Q What does it mean when someone is "going into shock"?

A Shock is the body's response to sudden blood loss, which most often occurs as a result of a trauma. When the loss of blood is substantial, the pulse rate increases and blood pressure falls. Blood is sent to the two main critical areas, the brain and the heart, and the supply to the rest of the body is extremely low. If blood loss is stopped and the victim is treated quickly with intravenous fluids and, if necessary, blood transfusions, shock can be reversed before there is damage to the vital organs or the patient dies.

552

Q What can be done to help motion sickness?

A Focusing on a stable, distant horizon can sometimes lessen the effect of motion on the inner ear that causes the motion sickness sensation. The antihistamine Dramamine is available over the counter but can cause drowsiness. A new alternative medication, meclizine, is now available over the counter. Both are effective if taken prior to the actual onset of nausea. The products do not work if the patient is already vomiting. A scopolamine skin patch, which is worn behind the ear, is an effective way to treat motion sickness. These patches are sometimes not available due to production problems at the company. Your pharmacist can compound a scopolamine gel, which is rubbed into the skin behind the ear. Scopolamine can cause dry mouth and blurred vision in some people. Try it before you go on a vacation to make sure the side effects won't interfere with your trip.

Diagnostic Tests, Immunizations, and Antibiotics

553

Q Why would a doctor run an SMA-20 at a yearly exam?

A An SMA-20 is a biochemical profile that measures blood levels of many different substances. Abnormal levels may indicate diseases or malfunctions of a body system. Be sure to discuss any abnormal levels with your health-care provider. Mild changes may not be significant.

554

Q What is a glucose test for?

A Glucose is the primary energy source for all body tissues. High blood sugar levels may indicate diabetes. Less than normal levels may mean a woman has hypoglycemia. For a glucose level to be valid, the patient cannot eat or drink anything for six to eight hours before the blood test.

555

Q What is a BUN test?

A BUN stands for blood urea nitrogen. High levels of BUN may indicate impaired kidney function, urinary obstruction, dehydration, starvation, fever, or antibiotics in the system. Low levels may indicate liver disease, malnutrition, or excessive fluid intake.

556

Q What does the creatinine test indicate?

A This test measures kidney function to determine how well they can filter and excrete creatinine, a waste product of muscle metabolism. High levels of creatinine in the blood may indicate significant kidney disease.

557

Q What does it mean if a woman's uric acid level is high?

A Uric acid is a by-product of the natural recycling of the body's own cells and from the metabolism of certain foods. A high uric acid level is associated with gout. Decreased uric acid levels are found in some types of kidney disease.

558

Q Is there a problem if a test indicates high sodium?

A Sodium is one of the body's principle electrolytes. It is involved in water balance and in the transmission of nerve impulses. High levels of sodium may be due to dehydration, excessive salt intake in the diet, kidney disease, or congestive heart failure. Low levels may be due to loss of body fluids through sweating, vomiting, diarrhea, extensive burns, kidney disease, and excessive fluid intake.

559

Q What is cholesterol?

A Cholesterol is a fatty substance (lipid) found in nearly every body tissue. It is an essential building block of cell membranes, bile acids, and sex hormones. High blood cholesterol levels are associated with the development of atherosclerosis, a condition in which the arteries that supply blood to the tissues are narrowed or blocked. If the vessels to the heart are damaged by cholesterol buildup, the diagnosis is coronary heart disease.

560

Q What's the good and bad cholesterol we hear about?

A HDL is the good cholesterol. This actually removes the cholesterol from the arteries and transports it to the liver where it can be eliminated from the body. LDL is the bad cholesterol that blocks arteries and causes heart disease.

561

Q How can I know if I'm at risk for heart disease?

A The cholesterol risk ratio that compares total cholesterol to HDL is the best indicator of risk toward heart disease. The lower the number, the lower the risk. A 4.5 or lower is preferred.

562

Q What are triglycerides?

A This is another fatty substance found in the blood. These levels are often measured along with cholesterol. Elevated levels, in the absence of increased cholesterol, is an independent risk factor for coronary heart disease in women. Some people will have elevations in both cholesterol and triglycerides. Fasting for eight hours should be done before this test to achieve a true level.

563

Q What is bilirubin?

A Bilirubin is a brownish-yellow pigment that is a by-product of the breakdown of hemoglobin, the oxygen-carrying substance in red blood cells. Increased levels of bilirubin may be due to an increased destruction of red blood cells. A decreased excretion of bilirubin may result from hepatitis, cirrhosis, infectious mononucleosis, or from gallbladder or bile duct blockage.

564

Q What does the alkaline phosphatase enzyme do?

A This enzyme is found primarily in the liver and bone. Elevated levels may point to liver disorders such as hepatitis, cirrhosis, cancer, chronic alcohol ingestion, or blockage of the bile ducts. Levels are normally elevated in growing children.

565

Q What do potassium levels show?

A Potassium is one of the principle electrolytes in the body's cells. It helps maintain water balance and is necessary for the proper electrical condition in nerves and muscles. Abnormally high or low levels can cause the heart to beat irregularly. Some diuretics deplete the body of potassium. Supplements of potassium should not be taken without proper monitoring.

566

Q What is chloride?

A Chloride is one of the body's most plentiful minerals involved in water balance and the acid-base balance of body fluids. Chloride is one of the ions in table salt (sodium chloride). High values occur in severe dehydration and certain kidney and adrenal gland disorders.

567

Q What is the problem if a woman has high levels of iron?

A Iron is a component of hemoglobin, the substance in the red blood cells that carries oxygen. Iron deficiency is rarely a problem in active adult males. Women may lose large quantities of iron due to menstruation, pregnancy, or breastfeeding. Low levels of iron are associated with anemia. High levels are associated with a condition known as hemochromatosis, which runs in families and can cause serious health problems.

568

Q What does phosphorous do in the body?

A Phosphorous is required for both bone growth and energy metabolism. Calcium and phosphorous levels are closely linked to parathyroid hormone secretion. High levels of phosphorous in the blood may indicate diminished activity of the parathyroid glands, healing fractures, some bone diseases, and excessive vitamin D intake. Low levels are seen in alcoholism and vitamin D deficiency and may indicate abnormally high activity of the parathyroid glands.

569

Q What does a blood test show about calcium levels?

A Calcium is the most plentiful mineral in the body. It is essential for the repair and growth of bone and teeth, the transmission of nerve impulses, muscle contraction, heart function, and blood clotting. Elevated levels of calcium in the blood may be due to excessive secretion of the parathyroid hormone, cancer, or excessive intake of vitamin D, dairy products, or calcium supplements.

570

Q What do protein levels indicate on a blood test?

A About 7 percent of blood's serum, or plasma, is protein. Increased levels may be due to dehydration, disease of the liver, or increased levels of specific blood proteins such as globulins. Decreased levels may indicate problems with the kidney, liver, or intestines or the presence of severe burns.

571

Q What is albumin?

A Albumin is one of the two major proteins in the blood and is produced primarily in the liver. It helps keep the fluid portion of the blood within the blood vessels. When albumin levels decrease, fluid may collect in the ankles or the lungs. In some forms of kidney disease, protein is lost from the blood into the urine.

572

Q What does a globulin level indicate?

A Globulin, the second major protein component in the blood, has many functions. High levels may result from dehydration, vomiting, diarrhea, cancer, rheumatoid arthritis, and some infections. Low levels may indicate malnutrition, problems with absorption from the intestine, kidney disease, blood loss, or severe burns. If the globulin level is significantly elevated, the physician may order a serum protein electrophoresis to determine whether a specific globulin is being overproduced.

573

Q What is a CAT scan?

A A CAT, or CT, scan is a special type of X ray. The patient is carefully positioned on a special examination table, and a technician focuses the X-ray equipment on the area that needs to be evaluated such as sinuses, the brain, or the spinal cord. A computer is programmed to control the X-ray machine, which takes multiple X rays or "slices" of the area. After these multiple images are obtained, the computer can then reassemble the information to provide a complete picture of the organ or area being studied.

574

Q What is an MRI?

A MRI stands for magnetic resonance imaging. This type of evaluation does not use any radiation exposure. The tissues are evaluated using magnetic fields, which are harmless. MRI is an effective way to look at tissues inside the body. Some MRIs are tubes that tend to make people claustrophobic, but the procedure is painless. The patient slides into this tube

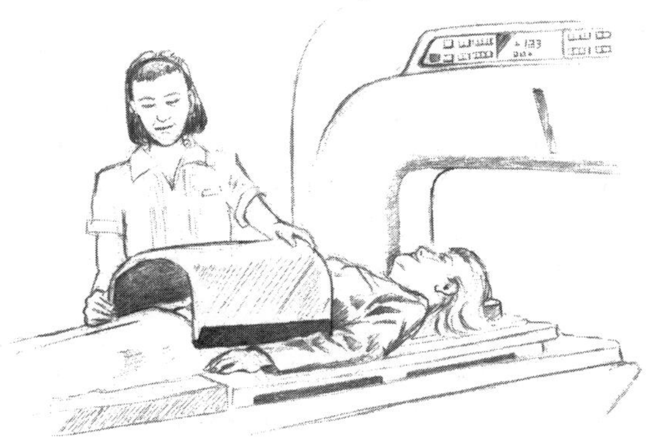

and has to be very still during the course of the procedure. Some facilities have "open" MRIs available. Since MRIs are expensive, they are usually only ordered when there is a clear indication.

575

Q What is an antibiotic?

A Antibiotics are medications used to kill or inhibit the growth of bacteria. It is important to understand that these medications do not treat viral infections. There can be serious and potentially life-threatening complications from this type of therapy. Therefore, antibiotics should not be taken unless necessary.

576

Q How and why do doctors take cultures for infections?

A A culture is done by obtaining a sample of the tissue or fluids from the area infected. A throat swab is taken for a sore throat and a urine sample for bladder problems. A technician puts the sample on a special culture plate or into a tube of nutrient media to encourage the growth of bacteria. Depending on the organism, colonies of bacteria may be seen the next day or it may take longer. The bacteriologist can then perform tests to identify the specific bacteria causing the infection.

577

Q Why does it matter what type of bacteria a person has?

A The type of bacteria needs to be identified in order to prescribe an appropriate antibiotic that will likely kill the infection. Without a culture, the doctor is basically guessing what antibiotic will treat the infection. After the bacteria has been identified and grown in culture, disks containing different antibiotics are placed on culture plates to determine the "sensitivities" of the bacteria to each different antibiotic. This information helps the physician in antibiotic selection.

578

Q What is penicillin?

A Penicillin was originally found as a natural product from a type of bread mold or fungus. Many antibiotics have been discovered as naturally occurring products from fungi. Penicillin actually kills bacteria while some other antibiotics just decrease growth rate. There are a variety of penicillin-derived drugs such as ampicillin and amoxicillin that kill many more types of bacteria than plain penicillin.

579

Q What are tetracyclines?

A There are many different drugs that are a part of the tetracycline family, such as doxycycline. Tetracycline's absorption, but not doxycycline's, is hindered by dairy products. This class of antibiotics is useful for treating a wide variety of bacterial infections, including bronchitis, chlamydia, gonorrhea, and mycoplasma infections. It is often used by dermatologists to help with acne. All of these medications cause sun sensitivity. Tetracycline after the second month of pregnancy can cause underdevelopment of tooth enamel and abnormal bone growth in the fetus.

580

Q What are the erythromycin drugs for?

A These antibiotics can be used in place of penicillin. At other times they are substituted for tetracycline. For example, erythromycin is effective in the treatment of chlamydia and acne. Zithromycin is an effective new drug in the family that is prescribed for fewer days of treatment. Nausea and vomiting are common side effects to these antibiotics but are less common with the new forms of erythromycin.

581

Q What are sulfa drugs?

A Sulfanilamide was the first antibiotic ever used. This class of medication is still important in the treatment of urinary tract infections. Bactrim and Septra are examples of the medications used for urinary tract infections as well as middle ear or sinus infections. Other than allergic reactions, side effects are rare. It is important to drink plenty of water to stay well hydrated while on this medication.

582

Q Why would cephalosporins be prescribed?

A These antibiotics are distant cousins to the penicillin family. Patients with a penicillin allergy may or may not be allergic to cephalosporins. One of the first drugs in this class was Keflex followed by Ceclor, Ceftin, and many others. They are used to treat soft tissue, skin, ear, sinus, throat, and lung infections. These drugs are well tolerated, have few side effects, and treat a wide variety of bacterial infections.

583

Q Are there any new antibiotics?

A Cipro and Floxin are a new class of antibiotics called fluroquinolones, which can kill a wide range of bacteria including some that are resistant to other drugs. They are helpful in treating resistant urinary tract infections, skin and bone infections, sinusitis, and pneumonia. These drugs have potentially serious side effects for pregnant women and young children.

584

Q Why are some bacteria resistant even to strong antibiotics?

A Medical science is trying to stay ahead of the microbes. Scientists thought they would be able to control bacteria completely when penicillin was developed. The indiscriminate use of antibiotics and the rapid adaptation of bacteria to antibiotics present a continuous challenge to the development of antibiotics.

585

Q What types of problems can occur from the indiscriminate use of antibiotics?

A Although antibiotics are wonderful drugs when they are truly needed, they can also have serious side effects. Some people have severe allergic reactions, even to an antibiotic they have taken in the past. In rare instances, an allergic reaction can cause sudden death due to anaphylactic shock (difficulty breathing usually followed by a loss of blood pressure). More common reactions include severe skin rashes, swelling, and severe itching. In addition, an imbalance of bacteria in the large intestine due to antibiotics can cause diarrhea, which may require hospitalization. There is also an increased risk of yeast infections in the vagina for women as well as, to a lesser extent, the mouth and the gastrointestinal tract.

Scientists are now identifying bacteria that are resistant to many, and sometimes all, antibiotics. This resistance has become more common as the use of antibiotics has increased. By limiting the use of antibiotics to specific situations, we can help ensure that they will be effective when they are truly needed.

586

Q Should a woman stop taking the medication she is prescribed when she feels better?

A Symptoms are often suppressed before the infection is entirely cured. If the entire prescription is not finished, the person may relapse or allow a stronger bacteria to survive. All medications should be finished regardless of how you feel.

587

Q How does an immunization keep you from getting a disease?

A An active immunization gives a person a weak form of the disease that it's trying to prevent. The immune system reacts to the harmless virus, bacteria, or toxin by making antibodies to fight it. The body has special types of white blood cells that can remember the information for a long time and quickly react if a real microbe becomes a threat.

588

Q What are the standard immunizations every woman should have?

A Women between the ages of thirteen and eighteen should receive vaccinations for measles, mumps, and rubella (MMR) unless they have proof of prior immunity. Most clinicians also recommend that women between the ages of thirteen and thirty-nine get vaccinated for hepatitis B by a series of three injections unless they are immune. A tetanus-diphtheria booster should be given between the ages of fourteen and sixteen, and women between the ages of nineteen and thirty-nine should have the booster every ten years. Women over forty should continue to take a tetanus-diphtheria booster every ten years, and women over the age of fifty-five should take the influenza vaccine annually.

589

Q Why doesn't anyone get a small pox vaccination anymore?

A Infectious disease experts believe this disease may have been eradicated from the earth except for a few cultures preserved in the laboratory. This is one of the great success stories in modern medicine. An immunization is not necessary because no one gets the disease.

590

Q Why do people need a tetanus immunization if it is rare?

A Although tetanus is an unusual disease, it is often fatal once symptoms occur. The immunization is almost 100 percent effective in preventing the disease and side effects are rare. Everyone needs a tetanus booster every ten years.

591

Q Is a hepatitis B vaccination necessary?

A Everyone should be vaccinated against hepatitis B unless she is already immune. The people at high risk are health-care workers, intravenous drug abusers, or those exposed to blood products. Hepatitis B can be transmitted by sexual contact. It can be a serious, life-threatening disease.

592

Q Who should take the flu vaccine?

A People who are chronically ill, are over sixty-five years old, or work in the health-care field should take a yearly flu vaccine. People with egg allergies should be cautious about it though, because the vaccine is grown in eggs.

593

Q Who should get vaccinated against pneumonia?

A Residents in chronic-care facilities or those who have a chronic medical disease, such as heart disease, diabetes, or renal disease, should receive the pneumococcal vaccine once. Other women who should get the pneumococcal vaccine include those with sickle-cell disease, Hodgkin's disease, alcoholism, cirrhosis, multiple myeloma, and those who have had their spleen removed. Revaccination for the pneumococcal vaccine is sometimes indicated in certain high-risk patients. All women over sixty-five should take the pneumococcal vaccine once, but revaccination is not generally recommended.

Contraception

594

Q Is the rhythm method a successful form of birth control?

A The rhythm method, also called periodic abstinence, is a successful form of contraception for a small number of women. This method of birth control is based on not having intercourse just before or during egg release (ovulation). A woman ovulates about fourteen days prior to the start of her period. She will ovulate on the fourteenth day in a twenty-eight-day cycle and on the eighteenth day in a thirty-two-day cycle. Because many women have irregular cycles, it is difficult to pinpoint safe days to have intercourse. The female can improve the reliability of this method by checking her mucus to determine when the egg white-like fertile mucus appears. It is important to remember that sperm can easily live for seventy-two or more hours in the female. Therefore, she must abstain from intercourse from day ten of her cycle to about day twenty.

595

Q Are vaginal foams effective against pregnancy?

A Contraceptive foams have a theoretical failure rate of only 3 percent when used precisely as instructed. The actual failure rate of about 20 percent is related to not using the product with each episode of intercourse. An applicator of the foam should be inserted no more than fifteen minutes prior to intercourse. There are no risks to this type of birth control except for the high failure rate and possible allergic reaction or irritation from the product. The foam may decrease the chance of contracting a sexually transmitted disease although we have little information about protection against AIDS. If a woman is not in a mutually monogamous relationship, a male or female condom should be used.

596

Q Is one type of male condom better than another?

A Male condoms are made from animal membranes, latex, and polyurethane. Condoms made of animal membranes are easily penetrated by viruses and offer less protection from disease. Latex condoms are less expensive and better barriers against sexually transmitted diseases. The polyurethane condoms are relatively new and produced for people who have an allergy to latex condoms. Male condoms are inexpensive, widely available, and don't require a prescription. This method of birth control has a theoretic failure rate of about 2 percent and an actual failure rate of 12 percent. The increase in failure rate is related to not using the condom all the time, rupture of the condom during intercourse, and not removing it correctly after intercourse. The condom needs to be inserted over the erect penis before there is any vaginal contact. A reservoir to catch the sperm should be left over the end of the penis. One partner needs to hold the condom in place on the penis while it is removed from the vagina. The condom is then carefully discarded. The effectiveness of the condom can be increased by using a spermicidal jelly or lubricant. Don't use any oil-based products such as baby oil or Crisco with the condoms. Women who choose oral contraceptives should use condoms too unless they are in a long-term, mutually monogamous relationship.

597

Q How does the new female condom work?

A The female condom is a relatively new product. It is also known as the vaginal pouch. It is a thin, flexible tube closed at one end. There are two flexible rings inserted into the tube: a large one on the open end of the tube and a smaller one on the closed end. The female or her partner squeezes the small ring and inserts it into the back of the vagina where it covers the cervix. The large ring stays on the outside of the vagina. The entire inside of the vagina is lined by the thin flexible tube. Sperm are trapped in the tube and never reach the female's tissues. After intercourse, the woman or her partner grasps the outer ring and twists the condom shut to prevent spillage of sperm. It is then removed and discarded. The female condom can be inserted prior to any sexual activity unlike the male condom. The female can control the entire process and be certain she is protected. The predicted failure rate is about 6 percent, and the actual failure rate is about 18 percent. This device is more expensive than male condoms but is also available without a prescription.

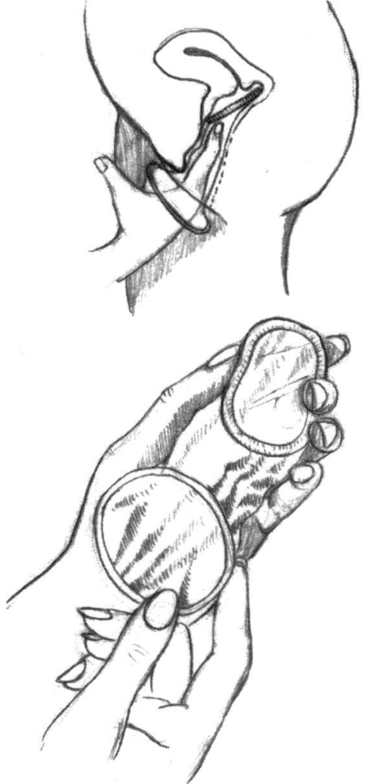

598

Q Can a woman be allergic to condoms?

A There has been an increased incidence of allergy to latex. If the male or female notices redness or irritation of genital organs after using a latex condom, try switching brands. If that doesn't help, try the polyurethane type of condom.

599

Q What is a diaphragm?

A A diaphragm is a flexible, dome-shaped latex cup that fits into the vagina and covers the cervix. It may be inserted up to six hours prior to intercourse and must be used with a spermicidal cream or jelly. It should be left in place for six to eight hours after intercourse to allow the sperm to be killed. The diaphragm actually works by holding the spermicide next to the opening of the uterus in order to kill the sperm. There is little effectiveness if the device is used without the spermicide. A diaphragm has to be fitted by a nurse clinician or physician. It comes in different sizes and is available by prescription only. The diaphragm should be replaced yearly and refitted if the woman gains or loses more than twenty pounds.

600

Q Is the IUD really dangerous to use?

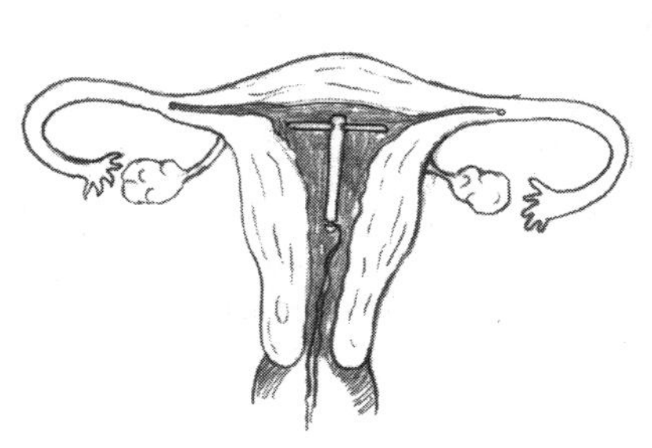

A In the early 1970s the Dalkon Shield IUD was found to have an increased incidence of complications, mainly pelvic infections. It was withdrawn from the U.S. in 1974. Many of the women who had these infections

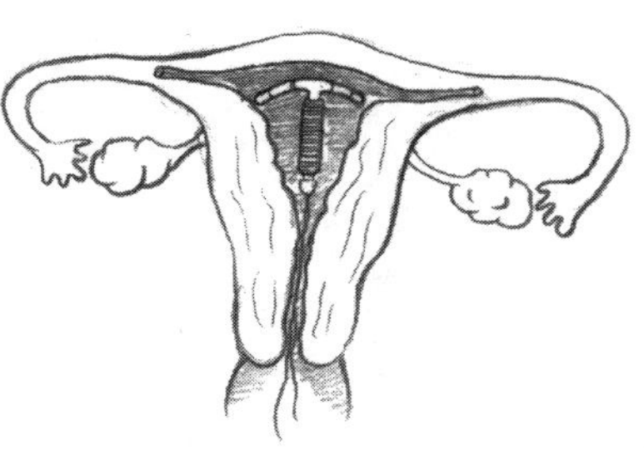

were unable to become pregnant due to injury to the Fallopian tubes. Because of the many lawsuits, many makers of IUDs removed them from the U.S. to avoid liability. There are currently two types of IUDs available in the U.S. An IUD should only be used by women who have completed their families and are in a mutually monogamous relationship. They do increase the risk of pelvic inflammatory disease.

601

Q How well does the IUD prevent pregnancy?

A The IUD is very effective with an in-use failure rate of 3 percent. Once it is inserted, the woman doesn't have to use or take anything. The Progestasert has to be changed at yearly intervals but the Paragard can be left in place for ten years. Some women experience cramps, spotting, or bleeding from an IUD but others have no problems. On rare occasions, the IUD will perforate or go through the wall of the uterus and damage other organs. The woman can check to see that the IUD is in the right location by feeling the small string that is left in the opening of the mouth of the uterus after insertion.

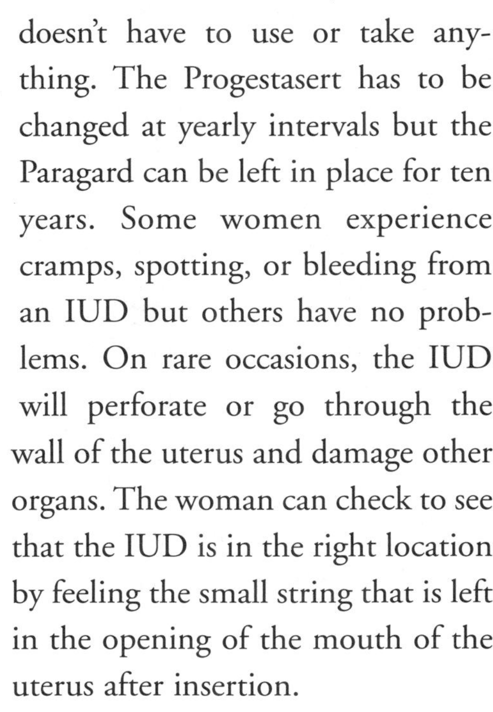

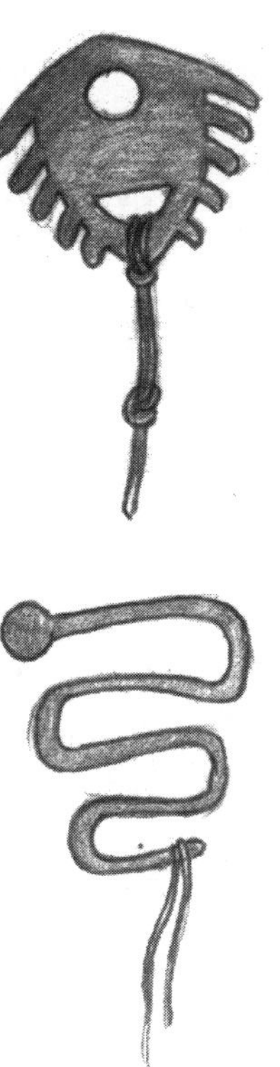

602

Q How is the IUD inserted?

A An IUD is usually inserted by a physician or a specially trained nurse clinician. It may be inserted at mid cycle or after the start of menses in the doctor's office. The mouth of the uterus is cleansed, and the IUD is gently inserted. The woman may experience some cramping and bleeding. A physician should be called if there is any fever, excessive pain, or substantial bleeding.

603

Q What is the injection that can be used for birth control?

A Depo-Provera is a long-acting, injectable, synthetic progestin that is extremely effective in preventing pregnancy. The failure rate is less than 1 percent. The injection is given every three months.

604

Q Are there side effects to the birth control injection?

A Most women experience some irregular bleeding during the first year of use. Within one to two years of use, many women stop having periods. The effects of Depo-Provera are reversible, but occasionally it requires more than a year for a woman's body to return to normal. In addition, women tend to gain an average of three and a half pounds a year while on the medication. This may be a major disadvantage to women with weight problems. Some women also complain of depression while using the medication.

605

Q Are the birth control implants that go under the skin still on the market?

A The Norplant system has been available in the United States since 1990 and is an effective form of contraception. With a local anesthetic, six matchstick-sized capsules are inserted under the skin, usually in the arm. These implants slowly release a synthetic form of progesterone and provide birth control for up to five years. The failure rate is about 1 percent. The most frequent complications are irregular bleeding and weight gain. The patient has to be willing to accept up to one hundred days of bleeding during the first year of use. The bleeding often improves after the first year. Some women experience increased breast tenderness, acne, and depression. After five years, or if the woman decides she wants to become pregnant, the implants are removed. Sometimes the removal can be difficult. The woman has to be able to accept some scarring or skin discoloration at the insertion site.

606

Q Are birth control pills safe?

A Birth control pills are some of the most well-studied medications. Over the years, birth control pills have been improved to offer the same effectiveness with fewer side effects. They are exceedingly safe if taken as directed.

607

Q How have birth control pills changed since they were first introduced?

A The pills had 50 to 100 mcg (micrograms) of estrogen when they were first introduced in the 1970s and were effective in preventing pregnancy, but they had side effects including fluid retention and nausea. The estrogen dose has been decreased over the years, and most now have 35 mcg of estrogen. The lowest dose pills (LoEstrin and Alesse) have only 20 mcg of estrogen. They are just as effective for contraception as the old pills and have fewer side effects.

608

Q How many years can a woman continue to take birth control pills?

A There is really no limit to the number of years a woman can take the pill. Stopping the pill for a while has no health benefit. If a woman is healthy, with no added risk factors such as smoking, most physicians will prescribe a low-dose pill until the time of menopause.

609

Q Does everyone gain weight on the pill?

A Although the older and stronger dosages of the pill tended to produce fluid retention and, therefore, weight gain, the new, low-dose pills haven't been shown to cause this side effect.

610

Q Can birth control pills discolor your face?

A The older, stronger pills caused some brownish discoloration across the nose and sometimes on the forehead. This is less common on the new, low-dose formulations.

611

Q Why do you have to take the pill at the same time every day?

A It is important to take them correctly to keep an even amount of the hormones in the body. The hormone levels drop after twenty-four hours and may cause spotting.

612

Q Why would a dermatologist prescribe birth control pills for acne?

A Often a hormone imbalance adds to an acne problem. The ovaries may be making a little too much male hormone and the skin may be overreacting to it. When this happens, oil secretions increase and block the pores in the skin, which in turn increases break outs. Birth control pills decrease the amount of male hormone that is in a woman's system and stops hormone swings that aggravate break outs. Many women experience improvement after several months on the pill.

613

Q When should a woman take her birth control pill?

A Some women take their pill during the morning routine of teeth brushing and makeup while others do the reverse at night. The time of day is not as crucial as the consistency of the same time each day.

614

Q How do birth control pills protect against pregnancy?

A The hormones in the pill prevent pregnancy by stopping egg release (ovulation) from the ovaries. In addition, they make the mucus at the cervix thick and sticky. The sperm have a difficult time swimming through the mucus.

615

Q Does a woman have to take the seven placebos?

A The placebos, the seven pills without medication, are a reminder. That way the woman doesn't have to remember to start taking the pill again after a week off. Some brands of pills contain a little iron to help prevent anemia (low blood count). It's not important to take the placebos, but it is important to remember to start a new pill pack on the right date one week later.

616

Q Can a woman with a family history of diabetes take the pill?

A Women with diabetes in the family can safely take oral contraceptives. It is important to be under the care of a physician who will do regular diabetes screening. Weight control and exercise are imperative to help prevent diabetes.

617

Q What are a woman's chances of getting pregnant if she missed just one pill?

A Chances of an unwanted pregnancy are low if you miss one pill. However, take the pill you missed the next day. Take the regularly scheduled pill for that day twelve hours later. Then you'll be back on schedule.

618

Q Is it more likely that a woman will get breast cancer if she takes the pill?

A Most physicians agree that birth control pills do not increase your risk of developing breast cancer.

619

Q Why are birth control pills always started on Sunday?

A This schedule is for convenience only. Most women prefer to have their period during the work week rather than on the weekend. The active pills are finished on Saturday and menses will start during the week. Your doctor will work with you if you have a different preference.

620

Q Is it dangerous for a woman on the pill to experience mid-month bleeding?

A It is common to have some irregular bleeding or spotting while on birth control pills. The bleeding is inconvenient but not dangerous. The bleeding can be stopped or decreased by switching pill types. Some pills, such as Lo-Ovral, have a very low incidence of breakthrough bleeding.

621

Q Is it safe to start taking pills because of severe menstrual cramps?

A One noncontraceptive benefit of taking birth control pills is that it decreases menstrual cramps (dysmenorrhea). This is a safe and effective way to control cramps. They are often improved or completely relieved by taking the pill.

622

Q Can a woman take birth control pills for irregular menstrual cycles if she is not sexually active?

A A woman does not have to be sexually active to be placed on birth control pills by a physician. Birth control pills usually produce regular, predictable cycles if taken as directed. Since the pill is safe and has been well tested, it's a good technique for helping women achieve regular menstrual cycles.

623

Q Do birth control pills affect a woman's chances of getting a sexually transmitted disease?

A The pill actually decreases the chances of getting gonorrhea and chlamydia. The thick mucus in the mouth of the uterus produced by the pill forms a partial barrier against these organisms getting into the uterus. There is no protection, however, from AIDS, syphilis, or certain vaginal infections such as trichomonas. The pill should not be used as protection from sexually transmitted diseases. Limiting sexual partners, knowing a partner's prior sexual history, and using condoms are crucial until a woman is in a long-term, mutually monogamous relationship.

624

Q Why would a woman have a light period or only spotting while on the pill?

A The hormone combination in the birth control pill usually produces a thin uterine lining (endometrium). Since there isn't much lining to shed, the period is light. Women on low-dose pills may not have a period at all. This isn't dangerous, but the woman may worry that she is pregnant if she doesn't have a period. If this is a problem, a pill that produces a heavier period can be prescribed.

625

Q How old do you have to be before you can take birth control pills?

A Any female who has had a menstrual period can take birth control pills. Although most young women are not sexually active when they start their menses, the pill can be prescribed for regulation of cycles, treatment of menstrual cramps, or acne problems.

626

Q Is there an age at which you should stop taking the pill?

A New studies on the low-dose birth control pills indicate they are safe for many women all the way through menopause, which usually occurs about the age of fifty-one. The health of the woman is more important than her age. Some physicians will not prescribe the pill for women over thirty-five who smoke because they are at high risk for complications. In addition to smoking, women with diabetes, high blood pressure, history of blood clots, or other medical problems are at high risk.

627

Q What are the risk factors of taking the pill?

A Although the pills are safe, they do have some risk factors. The major risk in taking oral contraceptives is stroke. Women who have had a blood clot should not take birth control pills. In addition, the pill can increase blood pressure in women who have hypertension and can increase insulin requirements in diabetics. Because the pill might make a breast cancer grow faster, women who have had breast cancer or have a mass that hasn't been evaluated should not take the pill.

628

Q Is it safe to smoke and take birth control pills?

A Smoking while taking birth control pills definitely increases the risk of serious problems. Many doctors are concerned and will not prescribe the pill for smokers over thirty-five.

629

Q How can a woman determine which type of birth control pill is best for her?

A Working with a health-care provider to select the best pill is important. It may be necessary to try several before finding the one that best fits a woman's needs. The same pill is not the best for every woman. Some work better to improve acne while others work better at controlling breakthrough bleeding.

630

Q How can a woman control the nauseated feeling she sometimes gets the first few days of a new pack of pills?

A Some women experience nausea the first few days of a new pill pack because their bodies have to adjust to the estrogen level. A mild antinausea medication such as Vistaril can be prescribed for the first several days of a new pill pack cycle. Switching to a lower dose estrogen pill can be helpful in controlling nausea. Estrostep is a pill that starts with a lower estrogen dose to help control nausea.

631

Q What should a woman do if her partner doesn't want to use a condom?

A Any male who cares about himself and his partner will be practicing safe sex. If the man will not use a condom with one woman, chances are he hasn't used them with others. Refusal to have sex will not put a woman at risk for a life-threatening sexually transmitted disease but unprotected sex will.

632

Q What is the most effective method of reversible birth control?

A Undoubtedly, birth control pills have the highest effectiveness with the lowest risk. In addition, the pill offers noncontraceptive benefits such as decreased acne, decreased risk of ovarian and uterine cancer, and improvement in menstrual cramps.

633

Q Is there anything a woman can do if she had sex without using birth control?

A A morning after pill is available by prescription. A woman would take two tablets of an oral contraceptive such as Ovral and repeat the dosage twelve hours later. The treatment doesn't always prevent conception, but it is the most effective method available today.

634

Q What's the best form of contraception for a couple who doesn't want any more children?

A Many couples decide on permanent forms of birth control such as a tubal ligation for the woman or a vasectomy for the man. Although both procedures may be reversed, it is important to consider the procedures as permanent.

635

Q How does a couple make a permanent contraception decision?

A Both operations are safe, effective procedures to prevent future pregnancy. A tubal ligation carries slightly more risk for serious complications than a vasectomy. The tubal ligation requires a general anesthetic while a vasectomy can be done under a local anesthetic in a doctor's office. Women sometimes choose a tubal ligation because they want to minimize their risk of pregnancy regardless of partner.

636

Q How does the surgeon tie a woman's tubes?

A There are a variety of techniques used to voluntarily block the Fallopian tubes that will prevent pregnancy. Most women have a laparoscopic tubal. Under anesthesia, a fiber-optic lens system is placed into the abdomen through a small incision near the umbilicus (belly button) to allow the surgeon to see the Fallopian tubes. Another incision is made at the top of the pubic hair. The surgeon grasps the tubes, one at a time, and places a clip or special type of rubber band on each one to block it. Alternately, each tube is cauterized or burned with an electric current.

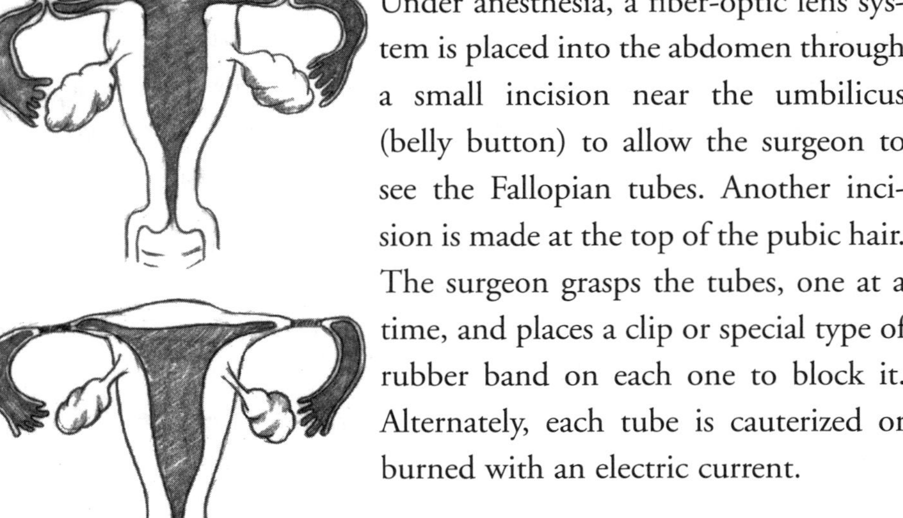

637

Q How does a doctor perform a vasectomy?

A A vasectomy is performed under a local anesthetic, usually by a urologist. Small incisions are made on each side of the man's groin area and sutures are placed around the tubes that bring sperm from the testes to the penis. The surgeon then closes the skin incisions.

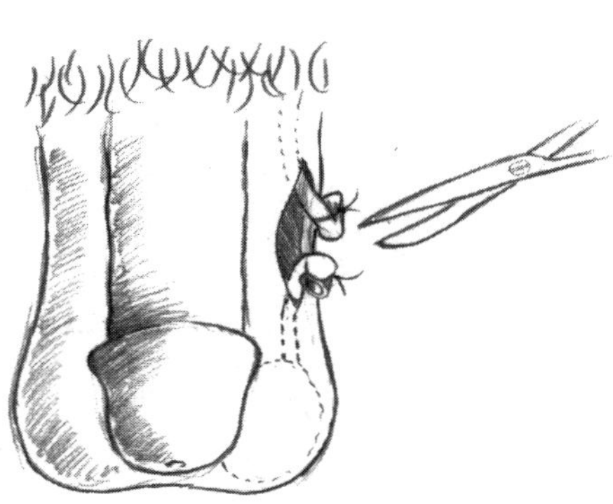

638

Q Does a man feel differently during sex if he has had a vasectomy?

A The male's hormones, erection, and sexual functioning are not altered by a vasectomy. The only change is the ability of sperm to pass from the testes out of the body. The sperm are very small and are absorbed by the man's body. Most of the fluid in the ejaculate is from other glands such as the prostate.

639

Q Why are some birth control pills different colors?

A Triphasic pills have several different colors of pills in the same package. They change the ratio of the estrogen and progesterone during the cycle to try to mimic the natural changes of hormones in the menstrual cycle. Monophasic pills contain three weeks of a fixed dose of estrogen and progesterone and one week of placebo pills that don't contain any hormones. There is no evidence that the multiphasic pills are better or safer than monophasic pills. They all provide excellent contraception if taken correctly.

640

Q What is the mini pill?

A The mini pill contains a synthetic form of progesterone without any estrogen. It isn't as effective in preventing pregnancy as the regular birth control pill, which contains both estrogen and progesterone. The pregnancy rate is 3 percent, compared with 1 percent from other birth control pills. You have to take the mini pill every day even during your period. There is some irregular bleeding on this type of pill and most women prefer regular pills. The mini pill is usually used only by women who want to use an oral contraceptive but can't take estrogen.

641

Q Is there anyway for a woman to change the day she will get her period if she doesn't want it to fall on a special occasion?

A The menstrual cycle can be shortened to three weeks or lengthened to five weeks to move a period by one week. A physician or nurse can provide instructions on how to change the menstrual cycle. Because hormone levels will be affected, pill schedules should not be changed on a regular basis.

642

Q How effective is withdrawal for birth control?

A Withdrawal is not a reliable form of birth control. Even before the man ejaculates, sperm-rich drops of fluid often spill from the penis. Sometimes the withdrawal is not timed right, and again, there is leakage. In addition, withdrawal does not offer protection from sexually transmitted diseases.

643

Q What should a woman do if a condom breaks during sex?

A Immediately insert an applicator full of spermicide into the vagina after a condom breaks. It's a good idea to keep a supply of foam around as a backup for this type of problem. There is a risk of pregnancy or sexually transmitted disease, but the foam helps to lessen the chance. You might also want to see your doctor about getting a morning after pill.

644

Q What should a woman do if she's had intercourse without a condom and thinks she has an STD?

A Talk with a health professional who is trained to deal with these types of problems. It may be embarrassing to discuss, but an untreated, sexually transmitted disease can be life threatening. A health-care professional can offer testing and counseling.

645

Q Will antibiotics interfere with the use of birth control pills?

A Some antibiotics will decrease the effectiveness of birth control pills slightly. Discuss an alternative form of contraception with a health-care provider when using antibiotics.

Termination of Pregnancy

646

Q What is an abortion?

A Termination of a pregnancy before the fetus can live independently of the mother is called an abortion. A miscarriage is technically called a spontaneous abortion. An elective termination of a pregnancy is a voluntary abortion or voluntary interruption of pregnancy.

647

Q What is a menstrual extraction?

A This procedure, sometimes called a mini abortion, is usually done in a physician's office as soon as the patient misses her menstrual period. The fetus is removed with a suction device. There is an increased chance that all of the tissue will not be removed when an elective abortion is performed this early.

648

Q What is a D and E?

A A dilatation and evacuation is a type of abortion usually done after the sixth week of pregnancy. This is most often a day surgery procedure that can be done under local anesthesia with sedation or general anesthetic. The cervix is dilated and the contents are removed. In early pregnancy, a suction device can be used to remove the fetal tissue. Later in pregnancy, fetal tissue may need to be extracted prior to suction or the scraping of the inside of the uterus to remove the remaining tissue. Pregnancy termination is safe if performed before the twelfth week of pregnancy.

649

Q Is there a nonsurgical pregnancy termination?

A Although available in the United States only through clinical studies in certain states, mifepristone (RU-486) is widely available in some countries. This medication can be used to induce abortion before the ninth week of pregnancy. The actual pregnancy loss is similar to a spontaneous pregnancy loss with cramping and bleeding. The procedure isn't always successful, and a physical abortion is sometimes necessary.

650

Q What are the risks of abortion?

A There are rarely problems from an uncomplicated, elective pregnancy termination. The most common complication of elective pregnancy termination is failure to remove all of the tissue. This may cause prolonged bleeding, cramping, or infection. Sometimes it's necessary to repeat a dilatation and curettage (D and C) to remove the remaining tissue. There can be excessive bleeding during the procedure, requiring blood transfusion. Rarely, excessive bleeding or damage to the uterus may force its removal (hysterectomy).

651

Q How does an abortion affect future chances of getting pregnant?

A Most uncomplicated elective terminations of pregnancy do not have an impact on the chances of a future pregnancy. If there is a complication from the procedure, such as an infection, the risks of problems with fertility increase. You should consider having a uterine X ray, called a hysterosalpingogram, if you don't become pregnant in a reasonable amount of time. This test determines if the uterine cavity is normal and if the Fallopian tubes are open.

Hormones

652

Q What is a hormone?

A A hormone is a natural chemical produced by a gland in the body. Most of the time, the hormone travels in the bloodstream to get to the target body tissues. For example, the hormone estrogen travels from the ovaries through the blood to stimulate thickening of the lining of the uterus.

653

Q What does the pituitary gland do in the body?

A The pituitary gland is a small structure located at the base of the brain. It is controlled by a part of the brain called the hypothalamus, which links the brain and hormone systems together. The pituitary is called the master gland because it regulates the hormones throughout the body: hormones that control the ovaries and reproduction, the thyroid gland, maintenance of milk production during breastfeeding, muscle and bone growth, and water balance.

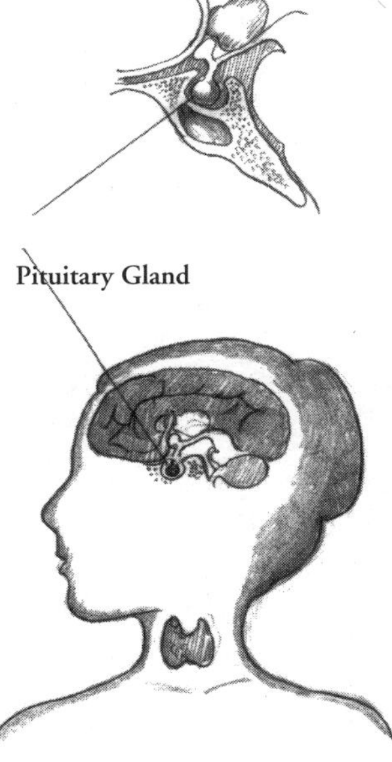

654

Q What is estrogen?

A The term estrogen really applies to a group of chemical substances that can stimulate the growth of the uterine lining. The most common natural estrogen in human females is estradiol, which is mainly produced by the egg units in the ovaries. Fat tissues synthesize a form of estrogen called estrone, and the placenta makes a weak estrogen called estriol during pregnancy.

655

Q Why is estrogen good for a woman?

A In addition to preparing the uterine lining for pregnancy, estrogen has many important functions. Estrogen keeps the lining of the vagina, part of the bladder, and the urethra strong and healthy; it stimulates breast growth and keeps bones strong, preventing osteoporosis; it improves the thickness of skin; and it protects against heart disease. New studies show that estrogen decreases the risk of developing dementia or Alzheimer's disease.

656

Q What causes the excessive facial hair on a woman that seems to increase with age?

A Hair follicles in both men and women are stimulated by the male hormone testosterone. The female hormone estrogen blocks some of the activity of the male hormone. As women age and their estrogen levels fall, the male hormone effect becomes more prominent.

657

Q What causes a teenage girl to have irregular menstrual cycles, acne, and dark hair on her face?

A Some women have a hormone imbalance that causes the ovaries to produce too much male hormone. This excess can cause increased facial hair. Birth control pills are helpful in controlling the hormone imbalance. Rare tumors of the ovaries or adrenal glands can cause similar problems. Consult a gynecologist to have hormone levels checked and clinical history reviewed. These problems can be controlled.

658

Q Why do women with a Mediterranean heritage have more body hair?

A Some women with this type of heritage have hair follicles that overreact to normal levels of male hormones and grow excessively. This is not a hormonal imbalance, and these women have normal menstrual cycles. This type of body and facial hair increase is called familial hirsutism.

659

Q What types of treatment are available to help with excessive facial hair?

A Birth control pills decrease the production of male hormone by the ovaries. By decreasing the blood levels of male hormones (androgens), the stimulation of hair follicle growth is decreased. This is a gradual process and takes three to six months to see an effect. A medication called spironolactone, originally developed as a diuretic, can block the receptor for male hormones on the hair follicle. Sometimes a birth control pill and spironolactone are used together. Once control of hair growth is achieved, electrolysis and waxing to remove the hairs is more successful.

660

Q Is it true that women have both male and female hormones?

A Both men and women have both sets of hormones. In the male the testosterone levels are very high and estrogen levels much lower. Conversely, in the female estrogen is dominant, but there are low levels of testosterone, the main androgen, and other mildly androgenic hormones. It is the balance of these hormones that is important.

661

Q What happens if a woman has too much male hormone?

A Women with polycystic ovarian syndrome (PCO) and some rare ovarian or adrenal tumors can produce too much male hormone (androgen). In severe cases, a woman can grow a full beard and experience balding. Her voice can deepen in response to the excess male hormone. Rarely, the male hormone will cause the clitoris, made from the same tissues as the penis, to grow (a condition called clitoramegaly).

662

Q Does waxing or shaving cause increased hair growth?

A There is no evidence that either will cause hair to grow faster than a normal rate. Hair feels coarser after waxing or shaving only because it is short and stubby.

663

Q Is electrolysis effective for hair removal?

A Many women find electrolysis helpful, but it is expensive and time consuming. Electrolysis is much more effective when hair growth is slowed with the use of birth control pills or spironolactone. It often takes three to six months of medical therapy to see a significant improvement in facial and midline body hair. It is also important to choose a well-trained professional to perform electrolysis.

664

Q Is there any reason why a woman would take additional male hormones?

A A small amount of male hormone taken with estrogen is recommended when menopausal women experience a decrease in sex drive or in natural aggressiveness. Solvay Pharmaceuticals makes a combination pill that combines estrogen and testosterone. This combination pill is called Estratest and also comes in a half strength formulation (Estratest HS). Not all women need to take additional testosterone after menopause. This deficiency is more common in women who have had a surgical menopause (the surgical removal of both ovaries).

665

Q Are there any side effects of taking male hormones along with estrogen after menopause?

A Although some may experience oily skin and acne, most women taking low-dose male hormones don't have any significant negative side affects. Deepening of the voice and hair loss are possible but unlikely. It is important to have cholesterol profiles monitored. Male hormones in some susceptible women can decrease HDL (good) cholesterol which could increase her risk of heart disease.

666

Q What could be physically wrong to cause a woman's heart to feel like it's racing?

A A fast heart rate can be attributed to anxiety, too much caffeine, a hot flush, too much thyroid hormone, or a heart arrhythmia. It is important to record whether the sensation of a rapid heartbeat is associated with faintness or weakness, the frequency of occurrence, whether anything seems to cause it, and if it coincides with a hot flush. Make an appointment to discuss the symptoms with a physician if it persists.

667

Q What is the thyroid gland's function?

A The thyroid gland is a butterfly-shaped gland in the front of the throat that produces a hormone that controls the rate of metabolism in the body. People with low thyroid have a slow metabolic rate, and those with too much of the hormone have a fast metabolism.

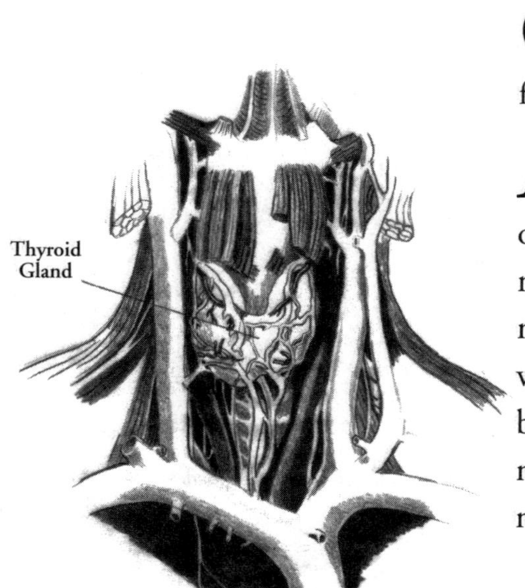

668

Q What are the symptoms of low thyroid production?

A Low or hypothyroidism is common in women as they get older. Symptoms include dry skin and hair, unexpected weight gain, fatigue, and occasionally menstrual cycle abnormalities. The TSH blood test measures the thyroid-stimulating hormone to evaluate the body's level. Depending on the test results, medications are available either to supplement the hormone or to decrease its production.

669

Q What causes a woman to have low thyroid?

A The majority of the time, a low thyroid is due to an immune disorder. The woman's body starts making antibodies to her own thyroid gland. Gradually, the antibodies destroy the thyroid tissue, causing a fall in the thyroid hormone production.

670

Q Is it safe to take extra thyroid medication to lose weight?

A Too much thyroid hormone can cause an abnormal heartbeat and make you feel anxious. Over the years, too much thyroid has been shown to increase the risk of osteoporosis. Women should only take thyroid supplements prescribed to treat a specific thyroid disorder.

671

Q Should a woman be checked if her mother has thyroid problems?

A As with many disorders, thyroid problems do tend to run in families. And women with a family history need to be aware of the signs of thyroid deficiency. Because hypothyroidism is so common in older women, a screen should be done when a woman is thirty-five and then repeated every five years.

672

Q How would a woman get her thyroid checked?

A Today there is a very sensitive and specific blood test to indicate whether any problems exist. Blood is drawn and a TSH (thyroid stimulating hormone) test is run. Fasting before the test is unnecessary. There is a strong relationship between thyroid hormone and TSH. The TSH levels will be high if the thyroid function is low.

673

Q What could cause a woman to feel pressure in her throat when she swallows?

A There are a variety of maladies that can cause the sensation of a "lump in the throat." Anxiety can cause the sensation and so can an enlarged thyroid gland. A throat examination should be done by a physician, preferably an ENT (ear, nose, and throat specialist). The doctor may want to have special X rays taken to check the esophagus and the throat.

674

Q What is a thyroid scan?

A A thyroid scan will be ordered if the gland is enlarged, has a nodule, or is functioning abnormally. Because the thyroid uses iodine to make thyroid hormone, the test will be done with radioactive iodine. This is a very low dose of radiation that is injected directly into a vein. The thyroid is then scanned to see how actively the gland takes up the iodine into its tissues.

675

Q Are thyroid lumps ever cancerous?

A Thyroid lumps are usually benign but can occasionally be due to cancer. Thyroid cancer is usually curable, especially if found early. A physician should palpate the thyroid carefully at yearly examinations to check for lumps. If a lump is found, a thyroid ultrasound, thyroid scan, and a biopsy may be done.

676

Q What is a goiter?

A An enlarged thyroid gland is called a goiter. Years ago, iodine deficiency was a common cause for goiter. Iodine was added to table salt for this reason. Today, iodine deficiency is rare and goiters much less common.

677

Q What's the best type of thyroid medication to take?

A Most people take a chemically pure product called Synthroid. Although it is available, it's not suggested that Synthroid be taken in a generic form. Generic thyroid medications tend to vary too much in potency to safely stabilize blood levels.

678

Q How often should a woman have her levels checked if she takes thyroid medications?

A A blood test is often done every six weeks at the start of the process to make sure the levels are correct. Because requirements for this hormone often change as a woman gets older, thyroid levels should be checked at least on a yearly basis.

679

Q Could a woman have a thyroid problem if she's very nervous, thin, and can't tolerate heat?

A Too much thyroid speeds up the metabolism and often causes weight loss. Women with hyperthyroidism are anxious and have an elevated heart rate, diarrhea, and a tremor. These symptoms warrant an evaluation by a doctor.

680

Q Can a high thyroid level be dangerous?

A Because the metabolism can increase, causing an abnormal heartbeat and body temperatures to escalate above normal, hyperthyroidism can be life threatening. This severe reaction is called thyroid storm and is more common during pregnancy. Immediate aggressive therapy is necessary to save the woman and her infant.

681

Q How is hyperthyroidism treated?

A An elevated thyroid my be treated by giving the patient a medication to decrease her response to the elevated thyroid hormone. This will lower the heart rate and ultimately decrease the metabolism. A different medication is available that can decrease the synthesis of thyroid hormone. These patients may eventually choose to take a high dose of radioactive iodine, which destroys the thyroid cells, or have surgery to remove the gland.

682

Q Can a thyroid problem cause a person's eyes to bulge out more than normal?

A The most common cause of an elevated thyroid is Graves' disease. This is an autoimmune disorder that stimulates the thyroid to make and release too much hormone. Another substance is produced by the same disease that increases the tissue behind the eye and pushes the eye forward. The appearance of the bulged eye is called exophthalmos and does not impair vision. The eyes may not regress even when the thyroid problem is under control. There are surgical procedures available by ophthalmologists to decrease exophthalmos.

683

Q What are the risks of taking radioactive iodine for a thyroid problem?

A There are minimal risks to having this type of radioactive treatment. It's important the woman not be pregnant or be around young children or pregnant women for about five days. The thyroid is so efficient at taking up iodine from the blood that essentially all of the radioactive iodine ends up in the thyroid.

684

Q What is parathyroid hormone?

A There are several small glands behind the thyroid that make parathyroid hormone. This substance removes the calcium from bones when necessary to keep the blood calcium level normal. Since a correct calcium level is needed for muscles to contract, including the heart, it is extremely important that the body regulate the calcium level. If one or more of the glands start producing too much parathyroid hormone, the bones will get weak as the calcium is removed and the blood calcium level will be too high.

685

Q Is there a hormone that can treat osteoporosis?

A Calcitonin is a hormone made in the C cells of the thyroid gland. It takes calcium out of the blood and puts it into the bones. The balance of parathyroid hormone and calcitonin keeps the blood calcium levels normal. Salmon calcitonin (Miacalcin) is now available as a nasal spray for the treatment of osteoporosis. Alendronate (Fosamax) is a medication that increases bone strength and decreases the chance of fracture.

686

Q What could cause a woman to produce milk in her breasts when she is not breastfeeding?

A Inappropriate milk secretion is called galactorrhea. It is most often caused by increased secretion of a hormone called prolactin from the anterior pituitary gland. Certain medications, such as birth control pills, some high blood pressure medication, and tranquilizers, can cause prolactin elevation. In addition, small benign tumors of the anterior pituitary can secrete prolactin. Any woman who experiences inappropriate milk secretion should see her physician, gynecologist, or endocrinologist.

687

Q How does low thyroid affect the production of milk in the breasts?

A The brain sends a message to the pituitary gland to stimulate the thyroid when production is low (hypothyroidism). It also stimulates the production and release of prolactin, the lactation hormone, at the same time. When the low thyroid is treated appropriately with Synthroid, all of the hormone levels go back to normal and the milk production stops.

688

Q What is diabetes?

A There are a variety of types of diabetes, all of which are characterized by higher than normal blood sugar levels. Insulin, a hormone produced in the pancreas, is necessary to move blood sugar from the bloodstream into the cells where it can be used for energy. There is an insufficient production of insulin in diabetics. Blood sugar levels go up and the cells of the body are starved for energy when the pancreas doesn't release enough insulin.

689

Q What are the different types of diabetes?

A Juvenile diabetes is the most severe and is called Type I. Patients with this type of disease have to take insulin injections. Type II, adult onset diabetes, usually doesn't start until after age forty. The tissues are resistant to insulin. Diabetics with adult onset disease may or may not have to take insulin. Sometimes diet, weight loss, and exercise can control it. Gestational diabetes is developed during pregnancy. Many of the women who have this type of disease will develop adult onset diabetes when they are older.

690

Q If a woman's immediate relatives have diabetes, can she expect to get it?

A Diabetes, especially the juvenile type, is an inherited genetic disease. Obesity definitely increases the risk for adult onset disease. Also, family history increases the risk of developing diabetes in pregnancy. The risk for disease can be modified by achieving a healthy diet, exercise, and normal body weight.

691

Q Why does diabetes sometimes subside with weight loss?

A Increased body weight increases the need for insulin. The escalation of a woman's weight and fat tissue puts too much stress on the pancreas. In this case, blood sugar levels rise due to inadequate pancreatic secretions. Conversely, blood sugar levels drop back down as a woman loses weight.

692

Q Why would a diabetic need to have a foot amputated?

A Diabetes causes damage to the small blood vessels, which feed the tissues of the body. Because of this damage, diabetics have an increased risk of stroke, kidney failure, coronary artery disease, foot infections, damage to the back of the eye, and nerve damage to the hands, feet, and bladder. Because the tissues receive poor blood supply, it is difficult for diabetics to fight infection, especially in their feet. Gangrene can set in, requiring amputation to save the patient's life. Control of blood sugar prevents this kind of vessel damage.

693

Q Why do diabetics have a higher incidence of vaginal yeast infection?

A The glucose in vaginal secretions is elevated when the blood sugar (glucose) levels are elevated. The yeast grow quickly due to the increased sugar. Although women may have several yeast infections a year, recurrent infections that are difficult to treat suggest a diabetes screening. Diabetic women tend to have more urinary tract infections as well.

The Heart

694

Q Why do women have a lower risk of heart disease than men?

A Because of the positive effects of estrogen, premenopausal women have a much lower risk of heart disease than men do. Estrogen increase the production of HDL (good) cholesterol. It is also a powerful antioxidant and has a direct effect on blood vessels to prevent hardening of the arteries (atherosclerosis). After menopause and the loss of estrogen, women quickly catch up with men for risk of heart disease. The replacement of estrogen continues to have a positive effect on cholesterol levels and blood vessels.

695

Q What is an electrocardiogram?

A An electrocardiogram is a test that checks the rate and rhythm of your heartbeat. There are portable monitors, called Holter monitors, people can wear to give their physicians a "real life" view of their heart rate and rhythm during daily activities rather than performing the test in an office.

696

Q Why do some women feel as if they have indigestion when they are actually having a heart attack?

A Heart disease symptoms seem to be very different in men and women. Females tend to have subtle and unusual symptoms. The chest heaviness and pain down the left arm that men typically experience are less likely to occur when a woman has heart disease. Women may experience sensations they interpret as stomach problems, a muscle spasm in the chest wall, or some type of menopause symptom. Any recurrent chest symptoms, especially associated with stress or exercise, should be carefully evaluated by a physician.

697

Q What are the causes of chest pain?

A The chest is a complicated structure and any part of it can cause pain or discomfort. When the bones of the chest, particularly the ribs, become inflamed it's called costochondritis. Pleurisy, chest pain when inhaling, occurs when the lining of the chest is inflamed due to a lung infection. Inflammation of the covering of the heart, the pericardium, is usually due to a viral infection and is also extremely painful. Pain from an infected gallbladder can have referred pain to the right of the chest or the right shoulder. Shingles, a recurrence of the chicken pox virus, is also painful and follows the pattern of a nerve root on the chest. Of course, chest pain can also be due to heart disease or reflux of stomach acid into the esophagus. Because chest pain is so complicated, a woman should see her physician for any recurrent or persistent pain.

698

Q What is a stress test?

A During a stress test the patient exercises to increase the activity of the heart while being monitored. Studies have shown that an echocardiogram, using ultrasound to monitor the heart, may be more accurate for women than the electrocardiogram (EKG). Any cardiac irregularities or signs of oxygen deprivation will need additional evaluation.

699

Q When should a woman have a stress test?

A Women should seriously consider a stress test if they are experiencing chest symptoms, have diabetes, high blood pressure, an abnormal cholesterol profile, or have a strong family history of heart disease. Discuss the possible need for a stress test with your family physician or consult an internist or cardiologist. A stress test can also measure your fitness level.

700

Q How does smoking affect the heart?

A Smoking adds about ten years to the risk of heart disease. If a woman is fifty years old and smokes, her risk of heart problems is comparable to that of a sixty-year-old woman. Smoking tobacco directly ages the blood vessels. The more you smoke, the worse the effect.

701

Q Does heart disease run in families?

A The risk of heart disease definitely runs in families. Looking at the family history of early heart attacks, abnormal cholesterol profiles, high blood pressure, diabetes, and unexplained deaths are factors assessed in determining a woman's future risk of heart disease. Women in the same family generally get heart disease an average of ten years later than the men in the family. Also remember that you can improve your risk with a healthy lifestyle.

702

Q What should a woman do if her cholesterol stays above two hundred regardless of how hard she exercises and watches her diet?

A A total cholesterol above two hundred isn't necessarily a bad level. It's the ratio of total cholesterol to the HDL (good cholesterol) that is the best indicator of cardiac risk. If the triglycerides are normal and the cardiac risk ratio is low, then there isn't a problem. If the cardiac risk is in the high-risk group, medication may be warranted to control the cholesterol level. These medications are successful in improving cholesterol and have been shown to prevent heart attacks. Some studies suggest that diet and exercise can only alter cholesterol by 5 to 10 percent.

703

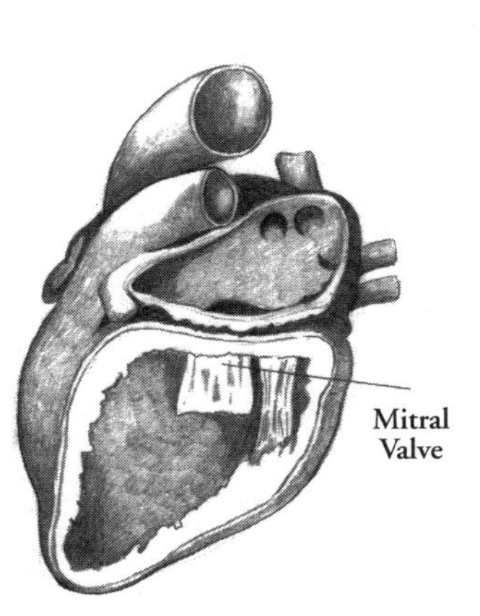

Q What is mitral valve prolapse?

A The mitral valve is located in the heart between the left atrium (filling chamber) and the left ventricle (pumping chamber). Sometimes, when the left ventricle pumps blood out of the aorta into the body, the mitral valve bulges and doesn't fit right on closing. This bulge is called a prolapse. If there is actual leakage, the condition is called mitral valve regurgitation. Mitral valve prolapse occurs in about one in twenty American women and is not heart disease.

704

Q What are the symptoms of mitral valve prolapse?

A Most of the time there are no symptoms. However, women can experience a rapid heartbeat or fluttering in their chest, fatigue, shortness of breath, anxiety, and chest pain. These symptoms are frightening if the cause is unknown. There are medications, called beta blockers, that are sometimes used to control the symptoms. It's suggested that women with this condition take antibiotics when they have certain medical or dental procedures because mitral valve prolapse may slightly increase the risk of a heart infection known as endocarditis.

705

Q How is mitral valve prolapse diagnosed?

A A physician listening to a woman's chest with a stethoscope may hear a click or murmur, suggesting mitral valve prolapse. Using an echocardiogram, which is painless and done with sound waves, the heart can be observed and the mitral valve checked for bulging or leaking.

706

Q What is a normal heartbeat rate?

A Heart rate is determined by age, fitness level, and the person's activity when it's measured. Normal resting heart rate can be determined by measuring the pulse rate for fifteen seconds and multiplying the number by four (to equal one minute). The normal heart rate decreases as the body ages. A woman should see her physician if a resting heartbeat is over ninety beats per minute.

707

Q How can a woman check her heart rate?

A There are two easy ways to check heart rate at rest or during exercise. One is to hold the nondominant hand (the one not used to write with) up with the palm to your face. Using the pads of the three middle fingers of the opposite hand, feel the pulse in the wrist area closest to the thumb. An alternative is to use the same fingers to feel on the side of the voice box for a pulse. In either case, measure the number of pulses in fifteen seconds and multiple by four to determine your heart rate per minute.

708

Q What is hardening of the arteries?

A Arteriosclerosis, hardening of the arteries, is a disease that clogs blood vessels, decreasing the normal flow of blood throughout the body. The initial problem is damage to the smooth internal lining of a blood vessel. Then cholesterol, white blood vessels, and scar tissue accumulate. As the condition gets worse, a plaque or thick plug can form, which slows the flow of blood and increases the chance of a blood clot that will completely block the vessel. When arteriosclerosis occurs in the arteries of the heart, it's called coronary heart disease.

Before the age of sixty, women have a lower risk of arteriosclerosis than men. Women with high blood pressure or diabetes are at extremely high risk for coronary artery disease and other forms of arteriosclerosis. Elevated total cholesterol, low HDL, a family history, high blood pressure, diabetes, menopause without estrogen replacement, and smoking all increase the chances of developing hardening of the arteries. Many of the risk factors can be controlled with lifestyle changes.

709

Q What does having high blood pressure really mean?

A Blood pressure is the amount of pressure the blood exerts against the walls of the arteries. It is determined by how hard the heart pumps, the elasticity of the walls of the vessels, and the size of the blood vessels. The small arteries (arterioles) in a person with high blood pressure are constricted, causing an increased resistance and forcing the heart to pump harder to move the blood through the body. Eventually the heart can get enlarged and weak, causing heart failure.

710

Q What are the symptoms of high blood pressure?

A Unfortunately there are no symptoms of high blood pressure until they affect some part of the body. It is important to have blood pressure measured at least once a year for this very reason. Readings should be done more frequently if a woman has borderline pressure readings or a family history.

711

Q What are the risk factors for high blood pressure?

A Although the most important risk factor for hypertension is a positive family history, smoking, diabetes, and being overweight increase a woman's risk. Decreasing salt intake helps some but not all people lower their blood pressure. Studies have shown that meditation and relaxation techniques temporarily lower blood pressure.

712

Q Why does a woman with high blood pressure need to have her eyes dilated and checked by an eye specialist once a year?

A The retina, the back of the eye, is one of the only places a physician can actually see the small blood vessels called arterioles. He is able to determine if high blood pressure is damaging the blood vessels. In addition, people with high blood pressure are at an increased risk for damage to the retina, which can lead to vision problems and even blindness. Keeping blood pressure under control with a healthy lifestyle and medication can prevent damage to arteries and decrease any risk of serious vision problems.

713

Q What is a stroke?

A A stroke occurs when the blood supply to the brain is interrupted either because a blood vessel is blocked or because it ruptures (a hemorrhage). One of the most common causes of stroke is atherosclerosis, which slows the flow of blood. Slow-moving blood increases the risk of blood clotting. When a clot is formed, the brain tissue that was nourished by a blood vessel dies. The patient will experience a loss of temporary or permanent function of that brain tissue. Blood clots can be formed in one part of the body and "thrown" to the brain through the circulation.

714

Q What are the risk factors for stroke?

A Strokes become more common as a woman ages. Prolonged bedrest and certain heart problems increase the risk of clots dislodging from the heart and going to the brain. High blood pressure, diabetes, abnormal cholesterol, and smoking all increase the risk of a stroke. Transient ischemic attacks occur when a woman experiences symptoms of a stroke that reverse themselves. This is a major warning sign that a stroke may occur. An evaluation by a physician should be performed.

715

Q What should a woman do to decrease her risk of stroke?

A The best step toward decreasing the risk of stroke is to make lifestyle changes. It's important not to smoke, be overweight, or sedentary. Blood pressure, blood sugar, and cholesterol checks should be performed on a regular basis. Also, discuss low-dose aspirin therapy with your physician.

716

Q Are there any vitamins that reduce the chance of heart disease?

A Discuss taking 400 IU daily of vitamin E with your physician. This vitamin has been shown to decrease the risk of heart disease about 30 percent.

717

Q What causes an irregular heartbeat in some women?

A Any abnormality in the rhythm of the heartbeat is called an arrhythmia. Many women's hearts occasionally skip a beat or have a minor palpitation, which is of no concern. However, some arrhythmias may be life threatening. Having an active eating disorder such as anorexia nervosa or having too much or too little potassium or calcium in the blood can alter the rhythm of the heart and even cause cardiac arrest. Excessive caffeine and nicotine can also increase the risk of a fast heart rate (tachycardia).

718

Q What is congestive heart failure?

A Congestive heart failure occurs when the heart is unable to pump as much blood as it should. The blood gets backed up in the body, depriving the tissues of adequate oxygen. Fluid accumulates in the tissues, especially the lungs (pulmonary congestion), and the heart literally fails to do its job properly.

719

Q What causes heart failure?

A Any disease that damages the heart can lead to heart failure. The two most common causes are high blood pressure and coronary artery disease. Women who have diabetes are more likely to experience heart failure because of the increased incidence of atherosclerosis and coronary heart disease.

720

Q What are the symptoms of heart failure?

A Fluid builds up in the tissues causing swelling in the lungs, legs, and around the liver. Fluid in the lungs (pulmonary edema) causes the patient to be tired and short of breath; the fluid bubbling sounds can be heard through a stethoscope. The patient may even cough up frothy pink fluid. Lying down makes the symptoms worse.

721

Q How does a physician treat congestive heart failure?

A A diuretic is given to help remove the excess fluid and clear the lungs. Administering oxygen, by mask or nasal cannula, helps deliver more oxygen to the tissues. The most important drug is digitalis, which improves the ability of the heart muscle to contract. The heart condition may be improved by treating the high blood pressure, or any heart arrhythmia, and optimizing blood flow through the heart vessels.

722

Q What is temporal arteritis?

A Temporal arteritis is an inflammation of the blood vessels found in the head and neck, although other large vessels can be involved. Some symptoms may include headache, scalp tenderness, and difficulty seeing out of one eye. Temporal arteritis is most common in women over sixty-five. The disease is caused by an autoimmune reaction that damages the blood vessels, leading to a decrease in blood supply to tissues. Untreated, blindness can result because of decreased blood supply to the retina at the back of the eye. A biopsy may be necessary to establish the exact diagnosis.

723

Q How is temporal arteritis treated?

A Because of the severity of the disorder, prednisone or another steroid must be used to decrease the inflammation and suppress the attack of the immune system on the arteries. The steroids may be gradually reduced after the disease is controlled. It may, in fact, take several years to completely stop the steroid therapy.

724

Q Why would a doctor tell a woman to stop taking diuretics?

A Diuretics decrease the amount of water and salt in the body by increasing urine output. They are effective and safe drugs for the treatment of congestive heart failure and some forms of high blood pressure. Diuretics can be psychologically addictive when a woman uses them for water weight loss. Most diuretics deplete the body of potassium and can cause a serious electrolyte imbalance. Electrolytes should be monitored when a woman is taking diuretics.

725

Q Are there natural diuretics a woman can use if she feels swollen?

A Celery, cucumbers, parsley, asparagus, and lemon have all been used as natural remedies to decrease bloating and edema (swelling due to fluid retention). Drinking water also pulls salt out of your system as the water is removed by your kidneys. Remember to also decrease excess salt in your diet. Decreasing the amount of carbohydrates and eating lean protein (chicken, fish, salads) will temporarily decrease the amount of fluid in the body. Do not use the herbal teas recommended by health food stores. There has not yet been sufficient study of them to consider safe.

726

Q What causes the ugly varicose veins in my legs?

A Varicose veins are swollen, enlarged veins that often occur on the backs of the legs and inner part of the calves. They occur when the valves in the veins fail to prevent the backflow of blood. The blood begins to pool in the veins and stretch the vein wall. A varicose vein in the anal region is called a hemorrhoid. Varicose veins run in families and pregnancy tends to increase a woman's risk.

727

Q Is there any way to prevent varicose veins?

A There is no known effective way to prevent these types of veins. It may be helpful to avoid wearing tight under-garments, socks or knee-highs with a constrictive band, and standing for long periods of time. Routine exercise that helps pump blood up from the lower legs, such as walking and bicycling, may be somewhat effective.

728

Q Is there anything that will make varicose veins ache less at the end of a long day?

A Over-the-counter support stockings worn all day long may be helpful. Discuss the problem with a physician who can prescribe a stronger, custom-designed, elastic stocking that will put more pressure on your foot.

729

Q What does a doctor do when stripping varicose veins?

A There are two different ways of treating varicose veins depending on their size and location. With one technique, the small veins are treated by injection with a solution that collapses them and makes the walls stick together. This is called sclerotherapy and must be done by a physician with special training in the technique. Another procedure is to tie off the top of the varicose vein as well as the additional "feeder veins" and remove the dilated vein under epidural or general anesthesia. Having several veins removed is not a problem since there are additional routes for the blood to take back to the heart. The legs are usually elevated for several hours and then wrapped with elastic bandages after the surgery. The surgeon may also recommend prescription compression stockings for the woman to wear.

730

Q How can a woman get rid of tiny spider veins on the legs that don't hurt but look ugly?

A Spider veins are tiny superficial varicose veins. They don't cause any health risk but are often a cosmetic concern. These veins can be treated with a laser or injected with a saline or sclerosing solution through a tiny needle. Multiple treatments may be necessary and the veins can recur.

731

Q What is asthma?

A Asthma is a chronic disease characterized by temporary narrowing of the tubes that lead to and from the different parts of the lung. During an attack, the lining of the tubes to the lungs (the bronchioles) become swollen, narrowing the space through which air moves. Normal mucus becomes thick and blocks the tubes, which makes it difficult for air to move in and out of the lungs.

732

Q What can precipitate an asthma attack?

A Usually an asthma attack is triggered by a substance the patient is allergic to. However, sudden changes in the weather, smoke, or strong odors can start an attack in some people. A respiratory tract infection or a virus increases the risk of asthma.

733

Q What are the signs of an asthma attack?

A A patient with asthma appears in distress with shortness of breath, coughing or wheezing, or both. Depending on the severity of the attack, breathing may become rapid and shallow. She will experience a rapid heartbeat and breathing requires a lot of energy. If medications are not available, she should seek medical assistance at once.

734

Q How is asthma usually treated?

A There are over-the-counter medications that can be used for mild asthma or breathing difficulties. They should be used only if suggested by a physician. Asthma is a serious disorder and requires medical evaluation. There are a variety of inhalers, sprays, and medications that are used to open the airways of the asthmatic. In addition, there are medications that can prevent attacks. Avoiding substances that trigger an attack is crucial for management of the disease. There are pulmonary medicine specialists and immunologists who specialize in the treatment of asthma. Some asthma patients need this type of specialized care.

Diet, Herbs, and Vitamins

∞ *735* ∞

Q What does a woman need to know about foods and vitamins?

A It's difficult to determine what everyone should be eating. The rules about healthy eating are in transition. It is important, however, to remember that variety and moderation are the keys to healthy eating. Studies have shown that people who eat a variety of grains, fresh fruits, and vegetables are healthier than those who don't. Information on vitamins and herbs is constantly being updated. You should read and question before making any diet alterations.

∞ *736* ∞

Q What happened to the food groups we learned about as kids?

A In 1992, the U.S. Department of Agriculture replaced the four food groups with a food triangle. The foods at the bottom of the triangle (grains like pasta, cereal, and bread) should be eaten more often than those on the top (fats and sweets). Fresh fruits and vegetables follow grains, then dairy products and meat.

737

Q How many vegetables should we eat each day?

A It is recommended that everyone eat five portions of fresh fruits and vegetables on a daily basis.

738

Q Are fresh products better than canned or frozen?

A Fresh vegetables and fruit are always preferable to those that have been preserved. Some vitamins are destroyed by heat, time, or improper processing. Frozen fruits and vegetables, however, do not get overcooked and tend to retain their nutrition better than canned. Frozen vegetables also contain a lot less salt than canned ones.

739

Q What can a woman do to balance her diet if she doesn't like a lot of vegetables?

A There are no substitutes for fresh vegetables. Try to rotate and eat the vegetables that you prefer frequently. Try new ways to prepare them so it doesn't seem like repetition. Buy a juicer or buy prepared vegetable juices as a substitute.

740

Q What does "organically grown" mean?

A Organic produce is grown in cooperation with the earth. Natural fertilizers such as composted materials and mineral supplements are used to amend the soil rather than synthetic formulated fertilizers. Pesticides are not used at all. Organic produce tends to be more expensive. There is a great deal of debate whether organic fruits and vegetables are better for you than the nonorganically grown produce.

741

Q Are whole foods better than processed foods?

A Simple, fresh, natural foods are minimally processed and retain more of their vitamins and nutrition than foods that are processed. Processed foods tend to have more additives that may affect some people in the form of allergies.

742

Q How many meals a day should a woman eat?

A Numerous clinical studies have revealed that consuming four to six small meals a day maintains an adequate level of blood sugar in the body and is actually healthier than the traditionally recommended three meals a day.

743

Q Why should we eat more complex carbohydrates?

A Carbohydrates (such as in potatoes, squash, breads, pasta, apples, and oranges) are a basic energy source, low fat, and full of vitamins. Many people feel hungrier when they eat too many carbohydrates because of the sugar content. It is better to eat small portions of these foods more frequently to keep blood sugar levels stable.

744

Q Why should people with low blood sugar avoid eating sugar?

A Table sugar (sucrose) and other simple sugars are quickly absorbed and raise blood sugar suddenly. The body's response is to release insulin from the pancreas to drive the blood sugar into the cells. Some people have an exaggerated insulin response, which drives their blood sugar even lower. By avoiding sugar, the blood sugar levels remain stable.

745

Q What can a woman do to try and ensure a balanced diet if she eats a lot of fast food?

A It may be more difficult to eat a healthy diet from fast-food restaurants, but it's not impossible. Most offer salad and low-fat protein selections like chicken. Stay away from sauces and highly salted choices. Many restaurants, such as Wendy's, offer nutritional information about their foods.

746

Q What is a protein?

A Protein is one of the major building blocks of the body and is found in all plants and animals. Muscle is composed of primarily protein and water. Protein can be changed in the liver to carbohydrates that are used for energy. Protein is needed in the diet to maintain repair functions of body structures.

747

Q How much protein does a woman need?

A Protein helps suppress appetite and level out blood sugar. Too much protein, however, can put stress on the renal system to secrete metabolic waste products. A good rule of thumb is to eat at least six ounces of protein daily.

748

Q What is the best type of protein to eat?

A Animal proteins tend to be complete because they contain essential amino acids. Dairy and egg proteins are also excellent sources but often include fat. Plant proteins are good but have to be monitored to be certain essential amino acids are included. Vegetarians who do not eat animal or dairy proteins must substitute through beans, rice, lentils, and corn.

749

Q How can you tell how much fat or protein is in a food?

A The amounts of fat, protein, and carbohydrates in a food should be clearly noted on the package label. Lean meat, fish, and poultry are almost 100 percent protein. A woman must read and do research to learn about foods that are not purchased in a wrapper.

750

Q How much water does a woman really have to drink every day?

A The average person should drink an eight-ounce glass of water six to eight times a day. Women who live in very hot climates or exercise a lot should drink more. The body will compensate for additional water intake by producing more urine.

751

Q Are artificial sweeteners in foods safe?

A There is no scientific evidence that artificial sweeteners cause disease in people. Aspartame and saccharin are considered safe, but the effects of long-term use are not known. People who have PKU, a metabolism problem, should not use aspartame. Many people claim that artificial sweeteners cause headaches, irritability, gas, and short-term memory loss.

752

Q What should a woman do if she thinks she may have developed a food allergy?

A People can become allergic to a specific food even though they have eaten it for years. If you suspect an allergic reaction, try avoiding the food completely, in all forms, for ten to fourteen days. If upon reintroduction, you experience the same symptoms, you have a clear answer. Other tests for food allergies may be helpful but aren't as reliable as an elimination trial.

753

Q Is there something medically wrong with a woman if she's having trouble digesting milk and cheese?

A Many people lack, or have low levels of, an enzyme needed to digest the sugar (lactose) found in dairy products. If a woman is lactose intolerant, dairy products will cause cramps, abdominal pain, gas, and even diarrhea. There are low-lactose foods available for people with this problem. Tolerance levels for lactose get lower as a person ages.

754

Q What's so good about eating yogurt?

A Yogurt is a high-protein, low-fat food that contains a live culture of lactobacillus. This is the healthy bacteria that helps to keep the gastrointestinal tract in balance. It is important to check the labels of the yogurt to make sure it has an active culture. Because this is a dairy product, lactose-intolerant women must avoid it. Lactobacillus pills, however, can be taken on a regular basis.

755

Q Why would everyone in the office seem to experience a 4:00 P.M. slump?

A Loss of energy late in the afternoon may be related to the diurnal rhythm of the adrenal gland. Most of us can't stop to take a short nap, which is common in many countries. An afternoon fruit snack may help compensate for the feeling of low energy. Some women find a caffeinated beverage or a short period of meditation is helpful to renew energy.

756

Q How many fat grams should a woman consume on a daily basis?

A The optimum number of fat grams is based on the woman's age, size, and activity level. Although it's known that growing children should not restrict fat intake, there is discussion over how many grams adults should consume. The U.S. Dietary Guidelines recommend less than 30 percent of total calories from fat. Many scientists think a diet of 20 percent fat will further reduce the risk of heart disease and help inactive older adults maintain their weight.

757

Q How does a woman know if she's getting enough calcium in her diet?

A The average woman should have a minimum of 1,000 mg, and preferably 1,500 mg, of calcium a day. The average American diet includes 600 mg of calcium a day. A woman should add enough calcium supplement to have a total intake of 1,500 mg.

758

Q How does a woman decide which calcium is best for her?

A There are two forms of calcium that are most effective. Calcium carbonate (such as Tums) should be taken with food. This form of calcium is not absorbed well without stomach acid. This is not a good choice if a woman is taking medication to decrease stomach acid for ulcers or reflux. Calcium citrate (such as Citracal) is best absorbed on an empty stomach. Stomach acid isn't necessary for absorption.

759

Q Should women take a multivitamin?

A Additional vitamin usage depends on a woman's diet. If a woman is eating five servings of fruits and vegetables and adequate dairy intake for calcium, there is little need. Using a multivitamin, however, will stabilize levels of vitamins and minerals that are missed for the most part in the average diet.

760

Q Does chromium picolinate control the appetite?

A Many say chromium picolinate helps to control appetite and maintain blood sugar levels. There have not been any reliable studies done with women to determine the validity of these claims. The reports, however, do not show any serious toxicity from this product.

761

Q Is it safe to take DHEA?

A There has been a great deal of information about oral supplementation of DHEA to attempt to prevent aging, decrease the risk of cardiovascular disease, and improve quality of life by decreasing fatigue and improving a "sense of well being." Like many alternative medical treatments, the promises may far outweigh the actual results. However, several of the studies have been done by reputable investigators. The numbers of participants in the studies have been small, and the follow-up has been short. Before there is any definitive information on the benefits of DHEA supplements, long-term, randomized, blinded studies in large numbers of patients will need to be conducted.

762

Q Should everyone take vitamin E?

A There is enough information to suggest taking 400 IU of vitamin E daily. This vitamin seems to decrease the risk of heart disease in women by 30 percent.

763

Q Why do some women take a lot of vitamin C?

A Many people believe massive doses of vitamin C can prevent, and lessen the effects of, viral illnesses such as cold and flu. The water soluble vitamin is not toxic but large amounts can cause bloating and diarrhea. There are believers and nonbelievers in the vitamin C theory. Scientific evidence is not convincing that massive doses make a difference.

764

Q Should women be taking vitamin D?

A People in sunny climates don't need extra D. People in cloudy climates, with little sunlight on a regular basis, should take 400 to 800 mg daily. Too much vitamin D can be toxic so consult your physician.

765

Q Are protein or energy bars good for you?

A The products available are convenient and well balanced with a high calorie content. They fill a need if other foods are not accessible but should not be a substitute for meals.

766

Q Are powdered supplement shakes for extra body building protein safe?

A The supplements may contain too much protein for a safe, balanced diet. Although some trainers and body builders feel these shakes are important to build muscle mass, eating a healthy diet is just as effective.

767

Q Is it unhealthy to be eating eggs on a regular basis?

A Although eggs contain a lot of cholesterol, they are high in protein and low in fat. Eggs can be included in a balanced diet that rotates food choices.

768

Q How important is a low cholesterol diet?

A A low cholesterol diet is important for someone with an abnormal profile. Studies have shown, however, that diet is only one component of a comprehensive program to control cholesterol. Decreasing saturated fats is equally important. Everyone should eat a diet low in fat to avoid health problems and obesity.

769

Q What's the difference between the different types of fat?

A There are three types of fats found in food: saturated, monounsaturated, and polyunsaturated. Saturated fats are found in meats, eggs, and dairy. Many processed foods contain saturated fats such as coconut oil, palm oil, or cocoa butter. A diet high in saturated fat will cause increased levels of LDL (bad) cholesterol in the blood. Monounsaturated fats found in olive and peanut oil, avocados, nuts, chicken, and fish may help lower your LDL cholesterol level. Polyunsaturated fats found in corn, sunflower, safflower, walnut, canola, and cottonseed oil help lower your total cholesterol but may increase cancer risk. The best diet is generally low in total fat consumption. When you do add fat, monounsaturated fat such as olive oil seems to be the best choice.

770

Q Why is everyone talking about antioxidant vitamins?

A Pull apart the word antioxidant. You get something that sounds like it acts against oxygen. We need oxygen to live, of course. With every breath, it's pumped into the bloodstream by the lungs and delivered to cells; they need oxygen to fuel the body's activities.

An unfortunate side effect of this process is the creation of unstable molecules called free radicals. They're also produced by exposure to toxins such as cigarette smoke. Free radicals can damage the genetic machinery of cells, causing them to multiply out of control, which in turn raises your risk of cancer. The molecules can also spur cholesterol to injure artery walls, leading to heart disease. It's even possible that free radical assault on our cells and tissues is what causes aging. Antioxidants trap free radicals before they can wreak havoc. The body produces its own antioxidant enzymes, but scientists believe that as time passes these defenses get overtaxed. That's why researchers have been investigating compounds such as the vitamins and pigments in plant foods to see if they can shore up defenses and lower the risks of cancer and heart disease.

771

Q How would soy products be helpful for menopausal symptoms?

A Japanese women experience fewer menopausal symptoms than women in the West. Diet may be one reason for the difference. Many women metabolize soy products into a form of estrogen. The Japanese diet includes soy products. Although there is not a great deal of scientific information on the subject, women in the Western world are incorporating more soy into their diets.

772

Q Why do some women take a melatonin supplement each day?

A Several studies suggest melatonin may be helpful in treating insomnia or as a prevention of jet lag. Although no toxic effects have been reported for this hormone, we don't have enough scientific information to encourage indiscriminate use.

773

Q Which medicinal herbs can a woman count on?

A Herb researchers say slippery elm bark for sore throats and the laxative psyllium seed are two remedies that have proven safe and effective. However, with all herbal therapy, there is little complete scientific information. The potency, effectiveness, and safety of herbs are not monitored by the FDA so, until more scientific information is available, use all herbs cautiously.

774

Q What is chamomile?

A This herb (*Matricaria recutita*) is from the daisy family and contains oils that can prevent gut spasms. As a tea, it can settle stomachaches and relieve menstrual cramps.

775

Q Why are a lot of people taking Echinacea?

A Echinacea (*Angustifolia*, *E. purpurea*, or *E. pallida*) was used to treat infections before antibiotics were discovered. It mildly stimulates the immune system to improve white blood cell activity. It may ward off illness if used in tinctures or tablets at the first sign of a cold or flu.

776

Q Is there some type of herb that might help migraine headaches?

A Feverfew (*Tanacetum parthenium*) in tablets, capsules, extracts, or fresh might help to prevent migraines before they even begin. The properties in feverfew decrease the smooth muscle spasms in the walls of the cerebral blood vessels.

777

Q Why would a woman be eating ginger candy when she was going through chemotherapy treatments?

A Ginger (*Zingiber officinale*) is sold as teas, capsules, and candied slices. Its properties are helpful for motion sickness and nausea. Large doses of ginger may be toxic.

778

Q Why have some women started taking Ginkgo?

A Ginkgo (*Ginkgo biloba*) may improve circulation. In capsules, tablets, and extracts it is reported to boost short-term memory and alleviate headaches and tinnitus (ringing in the ear).

779

Q What is St.-John's-wort?

A St.-John's-wort (*Hypericum perforatum*) as a tincture, tea, or capsule can help relieve mild depression and may relieve anxiety and unrest. The olive oil extract can be used externally for the treatment of hemorrhoids. The only concerns about St.-John's-wort are its tannin content, which slightly increases the risk of esophageal cancer, and the possibility that it increases sun sensitivity.

780

Q How can you tell what fruits and vegetables are the freshest in the grocery store?

A Look for produce that has few blemishes and is not wilted or droopy. The stems of specific produce should look freshly cut and not brown or dry. Organic fruits and vegetables tend to look less than perfect compared with those grown with chemical fertilizers and pesticides.

781

Q Is it safe to eat the fruit with a waxy feel to it?

A Although the wax will not harm anyone, pesticides may be trapped under it. It is better to choose fruit without a waxy coating. All fruits and vegetables should be washed with soap and water before consumption.

782

Q Should we be eating the skin on fresh fruits and vegetables?

A It is healthy to eat the skin on produce. The peel adds some fiber to the diet and may have significant amounts of vitamins. It is important, however, to scrub the skin to decrease any pesticide residue.

783

Q What is a portion size?

A A portion of any food should about be the size of a woman's palm. This is a much more practical guideline than weighing or measuring food portions.

784

Q Is fruit juice as good for us as fresh or canned fruits?

A Generally, a lot of the fruit fiber or pulp is removed in the juicing process. Vitamins can also be lost. Although fruit juice fortified with vitamins is good, freshly produced juice with the pulp is better.

785

Q What's the best thing we can eat at night when we're hungry?

A Any snack low in simple sugar and low in fat is a good choice. Some claim a high-protein snack, such as chicken or turkey, at bedtime makes them feel more energetic in the morning.

786

Q What is peppermint good for?

A Used as a warm tea, peppermint can decrease gas, indigestion, and colic. It is the menthol of the tea that is the active agent. Peppermint is safe and may also be helpful for menstrual cramps.

787

Q What do women need to know about Ma Huang?

A This herb (ephedra) is an effective nasal decongestant. The principal active ingredient is ephedrine, which is a form of amphetamine used in traditional medicine. It is a strong central nervous system stimulant that may be helpful in asthma. Ma Huang has not been shown to be effective for weight loss. It does, however, increase blood pressure and heart rate and cause nervousness, insomnia, headaches, and dizziness. Side effects generally make this herb a poor choice.

788

Q What's dangerous about alfalfa?

A Large amounts of alfalfa seeds daily may decrease the formation of blood cells or activate an episode of lupus.

789

Q What is yohimbe?

A Yohimbe is an herb that people take as a sexual stimulant. It dilates blood vessels in the skin and mucous membranes in people. Although it has been shown to increase the excitability of the pelvic nerves in rats, studies have not been done with humans. This herb is available at every sex shop in Germany but can be dangerous. High blood pressure can result if the herb is taken with red wine, certain cheeses, liver, and decongestants. Anyone with high blood pressure, heart disease, diabetes, and kidney and liver problems should avoid the herb until medical research is available.

790

Q Does aloe really have healing properties?

A Aloe is effective for the treatment of minor burns and aids in healing. The packaged products that contain aloe may not be as good as using the fresh gel taken directly from a plant. The juice taken from the leaf is a safe and effective laxative.

791

Q How is garlic beneficial?

A Garlic may be safe and effective in decreasing cholesterol. It is reported to be as effective as baby aspirin in decreasing the risk of blood clotting and stroke. Garlic may also be instrumental in preventing stomach cancer. In addition, the properties of fresh garlic may mimic those in antibiotics. Fresh garlic can be squeezed or sliced into hot water or soup as possible protection when cold or flu symptoms are apparent. Further scientific study of the properties of garlic are needed to substantiate these claims. Talk with your physician.

792

Q How can ginseng help with stress?

A Ginseng is used to support health as a general elixir and stress reducer. Although the benefits of the herb have not been scientifically substantiated, it doesn't seem to have any toxic effects.

793

Q What is Don Quai?

A Don Quai is often prescribed by herbalists for menstrual cramps, irregular cycles, and menopausal symptoms. Large doses can cause a sun sensitive skin rash. Although women are taking and talking about the herb, there is little scientific evidence that it is effective.

794

Q Does coltsfoot help with a cough?

A This herb may be effective in decreasing coughing and bronchial congestion. It is, however, toxic to the liver and may increase the risk of liver cancer.

795

Q Is there any herbal treatment for diarrhea?

A Bayberry is used to help control diarrhea, but its high tannin content may increase the risk of esophageal cancer.

796

Q What is evening primrose oil used for?

A This extract may help decrease breast pain due to fibrocystic disease. Other benefits, such as the treatment of skin disorders, are less documented. The pure oil appears to be safe but cheaper brands may be contaminated with other oils that can produce liver toxicity.

797

Q Is comfrey safe and effective?

A Although many herbalists recommend comfrey as a safe and effective herbal therapy, it can be dangerous when taken internally. The leaves of the deadly nightshade can resemble comfrey and occasionally contamination will occur.

798

Q Does licorice help a cough?

A Authentic licorice seems useful in treating coughs and colds. Many throat lozenges include the ingredient. Too much real licorice can cause high blood pressure, tiredness, sodium retention, and heart failure. Licorice candies, however, contain a harmless licoricelike flavor called anise.

Depression and Thought Disorders

799

Q What is depression?

A Depression is a mental state characterized by persistent feelings of sadness, hopelessness, and apathy. Symptoms may range from mild to severe, including thoughts of suicide. Reactive, or situational, depression occurs with a specific life event such as a death, divorce, or loss of a job. An endogenous depression is not a reaction to an event but rather a biochemical imbalance in the brain.

800

Q What's wrong with a woman who just doesn't want to get out of bed?

A People who are depressed have difficulty initiating any activity. They often want to be left alone and will stay in bed for long periods of time. They avoid contact with friends, are not able to perform daily activities, and find no pleasure in life. A physician should be consulted for an evaluation. There are medications that can help alleviate the symptoms of depression.

801

Q Why do some women feel so unhappy when they really have wonderful lives?

A It's important for women to understand they have is no control over a biochemical, or endogenous, depression. This type of depression is a physical illness that needs to be treated by a physician. An endogenous depression is just as physical as diabetes or high blood pressure. Positive thinking doesn't cure diabetes and won't correct the biochemical imbalance of neurotransmitters that causes depression. No one should feel guilty because they need an antidepressant.

802

Q Does having a family member with depression increase a woman's risk?

A The tendency toward depression is inherited even though the genetic basis of endogenous depression is not understood.

803

Q Why do women experience depression more often than men?

A About one in three women will have a significant depression in their lifetime compared with one in nine men. The difference between the sexes is unknown. Female hormones, the stress of pregnancy, and keeping feelings to herself in order to preserve a relationship may all increase a woman's risk of depression.

804

Q Why would a woman start waking up in the early hours of the morning and not be able to go back to sleep?

A Early morning awakening is a symptom of depression. Many people who are depressed are exhausted at bedtime and fall asleep quickly. However, they wake for no reason between 2:00 A.M. and 4:00 P.M. and can't fall back to sleep. Adequate treatment of the depression will usually help correct the sleep pattern.

805

Q Why is it sometimes difficult for a doctor to diagnose why a woman is so tired all the time?

A People with depression tend to have a variety of physical as well as emotional symptoms. They often suffer from nonspecific aches, pains, and fatigue. Headaches, dizziness, and gastrointestinal problems are all common. People who have a number of complaints and fatigue should be screened for depression as well as other medical illness.

806

Q Why is a weight problem sometimes related to depression?

A A change in weight, either up or down, can occur with depression. Some women with serious depression may have no appetite, eat little, and lose weight while others experience an increase in appetite and eat compulsively. Depression also hinders an adequate movement or exercise program.

807

Q How can a woman recover from a mild depression without medication?

A A regular exercise program, scheduling activities with friends away from home, and good nutrition with fruits and vegetables encourages lifestyle changes that can improve the ability to cope with mild depression. There are several herbs, such as valerian and St. John's Wort that may help with mild depression.

808

Q Does menopause increase the chances of depression?

A Depression is more common between the ages of twenty and forty. In fact, the woman with the highest risk for depression is in her twenties or thirties and stays home with small children. Women who work have a lower incidence of depression than their counterparts who stay at home with young children. Women going through menopause are not any more likely to be depressed than anyone else.

809

Q What would cause a woman to constantly snap at her children and lose her temper?

A Depression often coexists with hostility. If a woman is not happy with her life and sees no alternatives, she may act out her conflict. This is a high-risk scenario for child abuse. Counseling and medication may both be needed to improve the situation. No job is more difficult than being someone's mother.

810

Q How do antidepressants really work?

A Antidepressant medications gradually normalize the biochemical imbalance that leads to depression. It takes six to eight weeks to see the effect of the medication. Dosages start low and are progressively increased over time until the woman is stabilized. This method also helps to avoid side effects from changing dosages.

811

Q Are the new antidepressant medications better than the old ones?

A The new antidepressants offer improvement over older drugs in terms of side effects. Problems with dry mouth, constipation, and weight gain occurred with the old antidepressants. The side effects of the newer drugs are milder and resolve quickly. The new antidepressants offer the opportunity to treat mild to moderate depression to improve the quality of life.

812

Q How does a doctor determine which antidepressant is the right one for a woman?

A It isn't uncommon for the health-care provider to try several different medications before the right balance is achieved. The woman should not be discouraged if it takes several tries before the right medication formulation is found.

813

Q Why do some women feel guilty that they have to take medication to control their depression?

A Woman are taught they can conquer anything with hard work and a positive attitude. This is not true, however, of a biochemical imbalance such as an endogenous depression. Only medication can correct the imbalance of neurotransmitters in the brain.

814

Q Are antidepressants habit forming?

A Overall, antidepressant medications are not addictive. Xanax (alprazolam), an antianxiety medication sometimes also used for depression, is habit forming.

815

Q Once a woman starts taking medication for depression, will she have to take it forever?

A Depression is often cyclical. It may come and go spontaneously like waves. Some women will have only one episode that needs to be treated with medication while others have to be maintained with the medication to prevent regular depression episodes. It is generally recommended that the medication be continued for at least six months to help avoid a relapse.

816

Q Are there diseases that can mimic depression?

A Everyone who is depressed should have a complete medical evaluation prior to accepting the diagnosis of an endogenous depression. A low thyroid, poisoning with heavy metals such as mercury or lead, and certain connective tissue disorders can have symptoms in common with depression.

817

Q Why do some women feel so sad and blue in the winter but feel normal and healthy in the summer?

A Many people are affected to a certain degree by the weather. However, some women have a recurrent form of depression during the fall and winter months. This problem is called seasonal affective disorder (SAD). People with this disorder often crave carbohydrates and seem to go into hibernation, isolating themselves from others. This disorder may be associated with lower light exposure, which may alter a hormone called melatonin.

SAD is most often treated with light therapy although it's not an approved treatment by the FDA. These people also respond well to antidepressants such as Prozac, Paxil, and Zoloft, which increase serotonin in the brain.

818

Q What causes a woman to worry all the time even when there's nothing specific to worry about?

A Feeling worried or anxious a lot of the time is called nonspecific or free-floating anxiety. Women with this problem are very uncomfortable and never seem to be able to relax. They have a vague sense of dread that something bad is going to happen. They appear to be irritable and impatient with themselves and others. This sense of anxiety may be accompanied by many different physical symptoms such as feeling the heart is racing, dry mouth, dizziness, not sleeping well, chest pain, difficulty breathing, and heartburn.

819

Q What physical problems can mimic anxiety?

A Because there can be many physical expressions of anxiety, sometimes patients are misdiagnosed and prescribed medications that are unnecessary. There are some medical disorders, however, that can mimic anxiety such as heart disease, elevated thyroid, and a rare tumor of the adrenal gland that can release large amounts of adrenaline into the system. A complete medical evaluation is important before an anxiety diagnosis is made.

820

Q How can anxiety be treated?

A Anxiety is most successfully treated by a combination of behavior modification and antianxiety medication. Xanax and Klonopin are both effective medications for the control of anxiety but must be monitored because they can be addictive. Patients should never stop either of the medications suddenly because there will be symptoms of withdrawal. Buspar, which is not addictive, may be best for patients with moderate anxiety.

821

Q Why would a woman be "up" with a lot of energy one day and "down" in deep despair the next?

A People who swing from too excited (manic) to very sad (depression) are bipolar, or manic-depressive. During the manic phase, a person will have unlimited energy, be restless, wild, belligerent, and make bad decisions. At other times, they experience depression, sadness, and hopelessness. People with this disorder never seem to experience moderate feelings.

822

Q Can people with bipolar disorder be helped?

A The use of lithium has revolutionized the treatment of this disorder. Patients who are manic-depressive are often able to lead normal, productive lives using the medication to control symptoms. Lithium blood levels have to be followed closely to make sure they are high enough for good treatment without causing serious side effects or toxicity. Only a physician with special training, such as a psychiatrist, should be prescribing this type of drug.

823

Q What is a panic attack?

A A panic attack is a form of anxiety that occurs suddenly and is intense and unexplained by other problems. The patient usually experiences overwhelming fear accompanied by marked physical symptoms such as rapid heartbeat, chest pain, dizziness, shortness of breath, and numbness or tingling of her hands, feet, and lips. If the person doesn't understand the cause of the problem, she will often go to an emergency room thinking she's having a heart attack. Hyperthyroidism can also cause similar symptoms.

824

Q How are panic attacks treated?

A Understanding the cause of panic attacks can help the patient deal more effectively with them. Some therapists think these episodes are caused by traumatic early life experiences and are the result of deep-seated fears. Some mental health professionals help to decrease the panic attacks by desensitizing the person to her fears. Xanax and Klonopin are both effective medications for the control of panic attacks but must be monitored because they can be addictive. Patients should never stop either of the medications suddenly because there will be symptoms of withdrawal. Buspar, which is not addictive, may be best for patients with moderate attacks.

825

Q What can be done for a woman who has panic attacks and is afraid to leave her house?

A About one in three people with panic attacks will develop agoraphobia, which is a fear of open places. These people are unable to be in crowds of people. The problem escalates from not going to a mall, a grocery store, or the movies to not opening the front door to get the mail. Intensive therapy, with gradual desensitization and medication, is necessary if these people are to live normal lives.

826

Q What is schizophrenia?

A A psychotic patient has lost touch with reality. They are unable to determine what's real from what's fantasy. This problem often occurs in a serious medical disorder called schizophrenia. This is a serious psychiatric disorder characterized by severely altered moods, behavior, and thoughts. People with this disorder have distorted perceptions of reality, including hallucinations, illogical thoughts, and paranoia. The major tranquilizers such as Haldol have revolutionized the treatment of this disease. Historically, these people were placed in mental hospitals their entire lives. By using medications and frequent outpatient therapy, most can be managed at home with hospital admissions, if needed, for acute stages of their illness.

827

Q Is a woman's risk of mental problems increased if she has a family history?

A Mental illness tends to run in families. If a mother or father was schizophrenic, for example, a child has a one in ten chance of having a similar problem. The risk to the general population is one in one hundred. Studies with identical twins who grew up in different places show that environment may have something to do with the onset of mental illness.

828

Q What is a hallucination?

A Someone experiences a hallucination if she hears, sees, or smells someone or something that isn't really there. The most common hallucinations in psychotic patients are auditory (hearing voices). Visual hallucinations are much less common.

829

Q What is post-traumatic stress syndrome (PTSS)?

A People who live through a traumatic event such as combat in war, natural disasters, or personal abuse may suffer from a sense of depression, isolation, and worthlessness long after the occurrence. Patients with PTSS need intensive therapy to help them live through the trauma and develop workable coping skills.

830

Q Should a woman worry about Alzheimer's if she sometimes forgets little things?

A People in general forget things when they are distracted and experience an insignificant loss of memory as they age. People with Alzheimer's have a severe, progressive loss of intellectual function that interferes with daily activities. There is no known cause for the disease, but there are abnormalities in the microstructure of the brain at the time of autopsy. There is a great deal of research being done on this disease.

831

Q Is there any way to prevent Alzheimer's disease?

A A tendency toward Alzheimer's may sometimes run in families. Although several genes have been identified that increase the chance of early onset, most cases seem to be random. Recent studies suggest that estrogen replacement therapy after menopause may decrease the chance of getting Alzheimer's more than 30 percent.

Part IV
Life Management

Alcohol, Drugs, and Other Substance Abuse

832

Q Is drinking alcoholic beverages good for you?

A Moderate use of alcohol may have some health benefit. Excessive use, however, can be devastating to a woman's health and life. Studies have shown that men who have two drinks a day decrease their risk of heart disease. More studies need to be done with women.

833

Q When an article says one drink, how much alcohol is it talking about?

A A drink is usually defined as five ounces of wine, twelve ounces of beer, or one and a half ounces of hard liquor.

834

Q Are some forms of alcohol better for you than others?

A In moderate amounts, red wine has increased benefits over white because it contains a fairly high amount of antioxidants. Studies indicate beer decreases heart disease risk, but consumption of hard liquor increases the risk of throat cancer.

835

Q Is alcohol abuse more likely to be seen in men?

A The number of women who are addicted to alcohol is increasing rapidly. One third of all alcoholics are women. Because this type of abuse is typically thought of as a man's problem, women are less likely to be diagnosed and offered treatment.

836

Q What women are at risk for alcohol abuse?

A Women who have a family history of alcoholism are at the greatest risk. Educated, Caucasian women also seem to be at a greater risk, followed by women who lack coping skills, have experienced abuse, and have poor self-esteem.

837

Q What does being an alcoholic really mean?

A People in recovery who used alcohol to cope with life's problems are considered to be alcoholics. Their usage may have affected their physical as well as mental health and made life more difficult than it would have been without the alcohol.

838

Q What are the symptoms of alcohol abuse?

A People who abuse alcohol use it in excess to cope with life and to change how they feel on a regular basis. The drinking may get to the point of temporary memory lapse, which is called a blackout. Most people will deny they have a problem with alcohol because they don't consciously see the extent of their disease.

839

Q What are the DTs?

A The DTs, delirium tremens, is a severe form of withdrawal from alcohol. People who develop this syndrome are abusers who stop drinking abruptly. The syndrome is characterized by seizures, hallucinations, confusion, and panic. The DTs can be fatal and must be treated medically.

840

Q How does alcohol affect the brain?

A Alcohol is a suppressant, or sedative, that causes a decrease in reaction time, impairs judgment, and lowers a person's inhibitions. Too much alcohol consumed too quickly can cause drowsiness and even coma. It is these effects that make driving an automobile so dangerous.

841

Q Do women react different to alcohol than men do?

A Because alcohol is absorbed into body fat, women tend to feel the effects of a drink faster than men. In addition, men have more of the stomach enzyme responsible for breaking down the alcohol in the body. Women, therefore, become more inebriated on less alcohol than men.

842

Q What is cirrhosis of the liver?

A Cirrhosis of the liver is a progressive disease that may result from alcohol abuse, chronic hepatitis, hemochromatosis, or other liver toxins. The liver becomes scarred and shrinks. The normal liver cells that are responsible for many of the body's metabolic activities are replaced by scar tissue. The patient will eventually experience liver failure and die if the cirrhosis becomes severe and isn't treated.

843

Q Does alcohol abuse increase a woman's risk for health problems?

A The health problems associated with alcohol abuse tend to occur at a younger age in women and are more severe than those in men. Cirrhosis is extremely common in women alcoholics. In addition, there is a higher risk of cancer of the mouth, throat, esophagus, stomach, and breasts. Peptic ulcers, osteoporosis, and malnutrition are also common.

844

Q How much alcohol is safe during pregnancy?

A The American College of Obstetrics and Gynecology has suggested pregnant women abstain from drinking. Even two drinks a day has shown increased risk to the fetus of low birth weight, premature delivery, and even mild neurological problems. As little as four drinks a day can cause fetal alcohol syndrome. One drinking binge at the right time in the development of the fetus could cause severe problems. This becomes an issue for women who aren't using effective birth control and could be pregnant for several weeks without knowing it.

845

Q What is fetal alcohol syndrome?

A Fetal alcohol syndrome may be the most common preventable birth defect in the United States. Symptoms range from mild to severe. Many babies are small and have irreversible mental retardation. Their heads are small, and they have abnormally small eyes, deformed ears, and a flattened nose. Other defects include heart deformities, abnormal hips, hyperactivity, and other learning disorders.

846

Q What is the best treatment for alcohol abuse?

A Women with an abuse problem are less likely to seek treatment than men. There are several options open to a woman once she is willing to look at her alcohol problem. The telephone book in every city lists hotline numbers to call for help. In addition, Alcoholics Anonymous groups are available to help a woman learn new coping skills in a setting of her peers. Counseling, in addition to a group program, is helpful. The Betty Ford Center and similar facilities around the country focus on life issues in addition to the abuse problem.

847

Q Why do women substance abusers have a higher incidence of AIDS?

A Women who abuse substances are more likely to engage in risky sexual behavior than their nonabusing counterparts. It is difficult for a woman to be responsible and insist on condom use or monitor sexual partners when her senses are altered. In addition, intravenous drug users who share needles have a high incidence of infection with HIV.

848

Q How does the use of drugs affect sexual satisfaction?

A Women will report an increased intensity of sexual experiences and feelings while taking a variety of drugs. Studies, however, indicate a decrease in sexual functioning due to suppression of the central nervous system. Apparently the sensation from the drugs becomes more important than the physical pleasure of sexual stimulation.

849

Q Can a woman become addicted to prescribed medications?

A Antidepressants are generally not addictive. Antianxiety medications, however, are often highly addictive. Some of the drugs used for anxiety, such as Xanax and Valium, work "too well," and health-care providers may prescribe them frequently rather than referring a patient to counseling or support groups. The antianxiety medications are excellent therapy for acute short-term disorders, panic disorders, and severe anxiety, but they are easily abused and must be carefully monitored. These medications need to have a tapering off process and should not be abruptly discontinued.

850

Q Why do some women become addicted to pain relievers?

A Chronic pain complaints are more common in women. And, there are different points of reference for severe or debilitating pain. Physicians may fall into the trap of prescribing medications too frequently for the symptoms rather than helping to look for the cause. No one wants patients to feel unnecessary pain. Whenever possible, non-narcotic, anti-inflammatory medications should be used for pain. If narcotics are necessary, they should be used for a short period of time and should be monitored carefully. If long-term therpay is needed, referral to a pain clinic is often helpful in providing long-term pain management.

851

Q What are amphetamines?

A Amphetamines, or "uppers," stimulate the brain. Users initially report increased awareness, decreased need for sleep, and less hunger. The classic drug in this class is methamphetamine, which was initially used as a diet medication. Tolerance to the drugs are achieved in two weeks. Then more is needed to maintain the feelings. Side effects from withdrawal include irritability, insomnia, anxiety, and increased blood pressure and heart rate. Phentermine is a mild derivative of an amphetamine that is less addictive and is used in the popular weight-loss diet pills.

852

Q What are the withdrawal symptoms from amphetamines?

A People who take amphetamines on a regular basis complain of fatigue and sometimes nightmares when they stop using them. Also, there may be additional depression and anxiety.

853

Q What are barbiturates?

A Barbiturates, "downers," were used in years past as sleeping pills, such as Seconal and Nembutal. There is a more effective generation of drugs used today that don't leave a morning hangover. Abuse of barbiturates is dangerous regardless of the type.

854

Q Are there withdrawal symptoms from barbiturates?

A The sudden withdrawal of barbiturates can cause seizures and death. It is important to be under the care of a physician during withdrawal. Other symptoms include anxiety, inability to sleep, and profuse sweating.

855

Q What does cocaine do to a woman?

A Cocaine is increasing in popularity as an illegal drug for recreational use. This drug gives the user a sense of increased alertness and feeling of well being. Overdoses can cause hallucinations, anxiety, confusion, agitation, seizures, and sudden death. People on cocaine can be dangerous to others because of the side effects.

856

Q What are the symptoms of cocaine withdrawal?

A Depression, confusion, irritability, and even seizures can occur from withdrawal. Medical supervision from cocaine withdrawal is important to avoid any of the serious consequences.

857

Q Does cocaine cause birth defects?

A Cocaine can cause a number of major complications, including stillbirths, if used during pregnancy. The baby could also show signs of cocaine withdrawal after delivery.

858

Q What are opiates?

A Opium was the first natural narcotic made from a particular poppy flower. It has been used for centuries as an effective painkiller and as a recreational drug. Heroin is a derivative of opium. The synthetic narcotics (morphine, Demerol, and codeine) are almost as addictive as the original forms.

859

Q What are the side effects from narcotic withdrawal?

A Sudden withdrawal of narcotics will cause insomnia, nightmares, shaky hands, nervousness, pain, and nausea. Withdrawal should be done under medical supervision.

860

Q Is marijuana really harmful?

A There is discussion in medical circles about the possible addictive qualities of marijuana. Occasional recreational use appears to have few side effects. However, chronic heavy use can cause apathy, impaired judgment, disorientation, hunger, confusion, and even paranoia. Abuse in men may cause decreased production of testosterone and lead to sexual dysfunction. No health benefits have been documented from marijuana use, but it may be helpful in the prevention of nausea during chemotherapy.

861

Q Are there withdrawal symptoms from marijuana?

A Sudden cessation after heavy, prolonged use can cause irritability, shaky hands, trouble sleeping, decreased appetite, and gastrointestinal symptoms such as nausea and diarrhea.

862

Q What is PCP?

A PCP, phencyclidine, is a dangerous drug that is not used for any legitimate medical purpose. It can cause a wide range of symptoms including hallucinations, confusion, poor coordination, euphoria, and apathy. Heavy use can lead to paranoia and violent behavior.

863

Q Is tranquilizer abuse a problem?

A This class of drug (Valium, Librium, Klonopin, Xanax) is extremely effective at decreasing anxiety symptoms. More women than men use and abuse these drugs. Using the drug to cope with everyday life leads to both a physical and psychological addiction. Tranquilizers should be taken for acute anxiety disorders and not for chronic, low-grade anxiety. These drugs should never be used with alcohol. Talk to your physician if this type of medication is being prescribed.

864

Q Does a person go through withdrawal from tranquilizers?

A It can sometimes take several weeks to rid the body of these types of drugs. Sudden withdrawal can cause serious side effects and even seizures. Gradual withdrawal under medical supervision is strongly encouraged. People often experience headaches, anxiety, and trouble sleeping when withdrawing from even small doses of a tranquilizer.

865

Q Do fewer women smoke than men?

A Smoking is becoming more popular among girls and women. In 1965, a peak year for tobacco use in the United States, about 50 percent of men and 30 percent of women smoked. A 1992 study showed that the number of men smokers had dropped dramatically to 28 percent while the number of women smokers dropped only slightly to 24 percent. Lung cancer is now the number-one cause of cancer deaths in women in some states.

866

Q How is smoking harmful?

A Cigarette smoking is the number-one cause of preventable death in the United States. The list of diseases that smoking increases is nothing short of astounding. Smokers have an increased risk of cancers, chronic lung diseases, heart disease, and stroke. Women who smoke are more likely to develop peptic ulcers and cataracts. In addition, smoking damages the small vessels that feed the skin, causing increased wrinkles.

867

Q Does a woman who only smokes a little have a health risk?

A Smoking one to four cigarettes a day increases the risk of death from cardiovascular disease. The low-tar and low-nicotine cigarettes do not help to decrease the risk of cardiovascular disease.

868

Q How does smoking affect pregnancy?

A Women who smoke show a higher incidence of spontaneous abortion or miscarriage. Infants of mothers who smoked during pregnancy have a greater risk for low birth weight, sudden infant death syndrome, cerebral palsy, and other forms of brain damage and behavior problems.

869

Q Does smoking affect the reproductive system?

A Women who smoke go through menopause about a year earlier than women who don't smoke, and they have an increased risk of cervical cancer. Additionally, some studies suggest infertility may be more common in women who smoke.

870

Q What is the relationship between osteoporosis and smoking?

A Smokers have a higher risk of osteoporosis. One research study showed estrogen replacement decreased the risk of hip fracture in nonsmoking women but not in smokers.

871

Q Does being around someone who smokes have any risk?

A Exposure to second hand smoke does have health risks. Children who live with smokers have a higher risk of ear infections and respiratory problems including asthma. Adults may also risk heart disease from prolonged exposure to secondary smoke.

872

Q Would quitting really help a woman who has smoked for several years?

A The increased risk of dying from heart disease is gone within one year after smoking is stopped. The risk of lung cancer, however, can remain for ten to fifteen years. Former smokers have a longer life expectancy than current smokers. People who have smoked many years can definitely achieve a benefit from quitting.

873

Q Does everyone gain weight when they stop smoking?

A People tend to gain five to ten pounds when they stop smoking. Although there is a small slow down of the metabolism, the weight gain is largely due to the use of food as a substitute for the cigarettes. If walking or another activity is substituted until withdrawal is completed, there will be minimal weight gain.

874

Q What effects can a woman expect to feel when she puts the cigarettes down?

A The severity of withdrawal symptoms is directly related to how many cigarettes were smoked each day. Heavy smokers will experience more symptoms than casual smokers. Nicotine withdrawal can cause irritability, impatience, anxiety, difficulty sleeping, and a change in bowel habits. The symptoms peak two to three days after withdrawal and become more tolerable two to three weeks later.

875

Q Are nicotine patches and gum really helpful?

A There are both psychological and physiological addictions to cigarettes. Using an alternate nicotine source allows a smoker to deal with the psychological addiction first. She must completely stop smoking to use the patch or gum successfully. Then she can gradually decrease her exposure to nicotine and conquer the physical addiction.

876

Q Can behavior modification help with smoking?

A Many smokers use cigarettes as a way to relieve frustration and anxiety. There are certain triggers that will perpetuate usage. Sometimes the triggers, such as a cup of coffee or a drink, will have to be avoided until the woman stops smoking. Participating in a support group will help to learn what others do in place of smoking.

877

Q What's the relationship between depression and smoking?

A Smoking is one way women deal with depression. If a woman shows signs of depression, counseling and a non-addictive antidepressant medication may increase her chance of quitting and improve her quality of life.

Skin, Hair, and Nails

878

Q What is the best hand cream to use for dry skin?

A Heavy ointment products such as Vaseline are messy but provide the best lubrication for extremely dry skin. Dermatologists often recommend products that contain alpha hydroxy acid, urea, or lactic acid, which is found in Nutraplus and Aquacare HP. Oil and water combinations such as Lubriderm and Nivea are also good choices.

879

Q Why would a women's skin look reddened as if she has a rash?

A Rosacea is recognized by inflamed, red skin with red spider veins across the nose. This condition is common in women with fair skin who are middle-aged or older. Lupus can also cause a rash and should be ruled out by laboratory testing. There are many other causes of a skin rash that may need to be evaluated by a dermatologist.

880

Q How is rosacea treated?

A Long-term antibiotic therapy seems to be the only effective treatment for this condition. Avoidance of hot and spicy foods and the use of sunscreen are important.

881

Q Is the cosmetic industry regulated?

A The FDA, or Food and Drug Administration, states a cosmetic cannot alter the structure or function of the human body. If a product or ingredient does alter the body, it's considered a drug and is regulated closely. The cosmetic companies are therefore self-regulated.

882

Q Is there anything a woman should know about wearing cosmetics?

A Cosmetics are a personal choice and generally don't improve a woman's health. Some makeup foundations do have sunscreens to protect skin from harmful sun rays. It is important to be a proactive consumer and read the labels. Remember to throw away mascara after six months to avoid bacteria that might cause an eye infection. It's also important to clean makeup brushes and applicators at least every other month to remove any bacteria that may develop.

883

Q Do vitamins applied to the skin really work?

A It is doubtful that any of the fat soluble vitamins, such as E and D, penetrate deeply enough into the skin to make a significant difference. However, some of the new high-potency vitamin C preparations may penetrate the skin deeply enough to actually improve it. Skin Ceuticals's High Potency Topical Vitamin C Serum is one such product and may encourage the production of new collagen, the repair of damaged collagen and reversal of sun damage. This product has also shown some promise in the treatment and control of rosacea. More studies are needed to substantiate the claims of this product.

884

Q Do cosmetics contain hormones?

A There are several products that include estrogen. There have been cases of breast development in young girls who used their mother's creams even though the FDA requires estrogen levels to be low. Remember that if a cosmetic ingredient significantly alters the body, it is called a drug and can't be sold over the counter. Ask for scientific evidence that a cosmetic works the way it claims to.

885

Q What does hypoallergenic mean?

A Hypoallergenic means the product does not contain chemicals known to have a high risk of skin irritation or allergy. There are no guarantees, however, that someone might not be allergic to some component of the formulation.

886

Q What is PABA?

A PABA, para-aminobenzoic acid, is an excellent sunscreen but is also a common cause of allergic skin reactions.

People who are PABA sensitive must find products that are free of any PABA properties.

887

Q Does Retin-A remove wrinkles?

A Retin-A works to smooth out fine lines in the skin by causing the skin cells to renew themselves faster, making the skin look plumper. There is some evidence that this product can reverse sun damage by producing more collagen. Collagen is the support structure for the skin. The product must be used for about six weeks before any visible changes are seen.

888

Q Are there any side effects from using Retin-A?

A Retin-A can cause redness, irritation, and peeling of the skin. A sunscreen should be used in conjunction with Retin-A products because the skin becomes sun sensitive. Skin improvements achieved with Retin-A are lost when a woman stops using it.

889

Q Why does skin wrinkle over time?

A The skin becomes drier and loses elasticity, due to the change in collagen, as it ages. It's difficult for skin products to penetrate the main collagen layer to really affect the skin's structure.

890

Q Why do some women have more wrinkles than others?

A Some women inherit better skin qualities than others. Women who are thin and have dry skin tend to get more wrinkles than others. In addition, sun damage and cigarette smoking speed up the aging process of the skin.

891

Q How can cigarette smoking damage skin?

A The nicotine and other toxins in the smoke damage the small vessels that feed the skin. Because blood flow to the skin is decreased, the skin looks older and is damaged more easily by sun exposure.

892

Q What does a moisturizer do?

A A moisturizer softens the top layer of the skin to help smooth out superficial lines. Moisturizers do not penetrate the deep layers of the skin. They do, however, help to hold water near the top of the skin. Drinking water is the most important factor in maintaining moisture in the deep layers of the skin. It's important to choose a moisturizer that doesn't clog pores or cause acne problems.

893

Q Are eye creams necessary?

A The skin around the eye is especially thin and easily damaged. Because sunscreens should not be used so close to the eye, sunglasses become a necessary screen. There is no scientific evidence that eye creams decrease skin aging.

894

Q What's the best way to clean my face?

A Gentle cleansing with a mild, hypoallergenic, nondrying soap is the best cleaning method. There are a number of products that will do the job without clogging pores. Cetaphil as well as Aveeno are good cleaning agents.

895

Q What causes the ugly dark spots on a woman's hands?

A These pigmentation changes are sometimes called liver spots. They are most common on the backs of the hands and face in people over fifty but may appear sooner. Despite their name, they are not related to the liver. No one knows what causes them. Sun exposure may be a significant factor.

896

Q Do liver spots increase the chance of skin cancer?

A Most dark spots are harmless and don't need to be treated except for cosmetic purposes. However, it is sometimes difficult to tell the difference between a skin cancer such as melanoma and a harmless spot. Any skin change that thickens, bleeds, grows, or changes color should be checked by a physician. Since people with liver spots may have had more sun exposure, they may be more susceptible to skin cancer.

897

Q What are the dark skin lesions that look like wax?

A These waxlike lesions, actinic keratoses, are benign skin changes but should be checked by a physician if they start to grow, bleed, get thick, or change color.

898

Q Can actinic keratoses be removed?

A The lesions can be removed by freezing (cryosurgery) or by using bichloracetic acid. Surgical removal may be done if tissue is needed to confirm a benign diagnosis. A plastic surgeon or dermatologist should be consulted if these lesions appear.

899

Q Are wrinkles related in any way to sun exposure?

A The sun's rays, especially the ultraviolet ones, penetrate the skin and damage the organization of the collagen layer. Preventing sun damage to the skin over the years can decrease the development of wrinkles by more than 50 percent.

900

Q Why should women wear a sunscreen every day?

A Much of the sun damage to the skin is "incidental." Daily activities such as getting in and out of the car expose a woman to the sun. Sunscreen applied daily can help decrease skin damage. Some cosmetic companies are now including sunscreen in their formulations.

901

Q Is sunscreen only for the face?

A Sunscreen should be applied to the face, neck, back of the neck, and backs of the hands daily.

902

Q What's the best way for a woman to protect her skin if she's planning a vacation at the beach?

A Sunscreen should be applied to all exposed skin areas for protection and reapplied every few hours. Hats and umbrellas are good protectors for both the skin and hair.

903

Q What type of sunscreen is the best?

A A number fifteen sunscreen is a minimum requirement for good skin protection. This number means that you can be in the sun fifteen times longer than someone not using sunscreen. You should probably avoid PABA unless you know you are not allergic to it.

904

Q Are all sunscreens greasy feeling?

A There are a number of sunscreens that don't have any oil in the formulation and won't clog pores or irritate skin. Check the labels for "oil free." Clinique makes a good oil-free sunblock in a pump spray can.

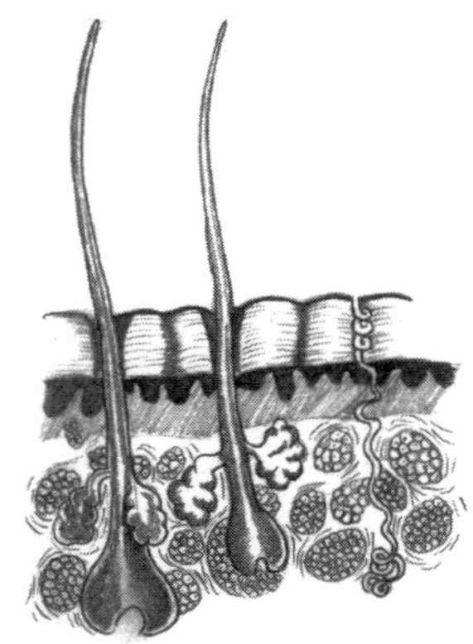

905

Q How does hair grow?

A Hair is composed of dead cells that grow from clusters of dividing, living cells that are under the skin. These are called hair follicles. As the follicle cells divide, they push up from the scalp and make the hair grow longer.

906

Q How fast can hair grow?

A Hair grows at an average rate of one half inch per month. There are over one hundred thousand hairs on each person's scalp. The average hair grows for about two years before it goes into a rest phase and falls out. If too many hairs go into a resting phase at once, the person's hair will, at least temporarily, get thinner.

907

Q What can a woman do to help her hair stay healthy?

A Good nutrition and a healthy lifestyle make a difference in the health of a woman's hair. In addition, hair needs to be protected from damage by the sun, wind, excess heat, and harsh chemicals. There are natural oils produced at the base of each hair that can be distributed to the rest of the hair by gentle brushing with a soft brush. Overbrushing may cause hair loss.

908

Q How often should a woman shampoo her hair?

A Hair should be shampooed as often as necessary to keep it clean and shiny. There is no evidence indicating washing hair too frequently is damaging. Use warm, not hot, water and a conditioner if needed. Treat hair gently because it is vulnerable to damage and stretching while it is wet.

909

Q Does it damage hair to use a hair dryer and curling iron regularly?

A The more processing a woman does to the hair, the greater the risk of damage. Daily heat processing treatments, with a dryer, curling iron, or hot rollers, will damage the protein in the hair. The hair is composed of dead cells that can't repair themselves. It's better to prevent hair damage than use surface treatments, such as conditioners, that mask the damage.

910

Q What causes women to have different hair color?

A The natural color of hair is genetically determined by the amount of melanin in the middle layer of the hair, called the cortex. Women with blond hair produce very little melanin in their hair follicles compared with dark-haired women, who produce a great deal.

911

Q Why do some women turn gray at a young age?

A Some hair follicles lose the ability to make melanin. The result is a colorless hair that has been called gray. The only color in gray hair is the reflection or opaque quality caused by the protein in the different layers. The age at which a woman turns gray is genetically determined and has nothing to do with general health.

912

Q What makes hair straight or curly?

A The shape of the hair's cortex is genetically determined and indicates whether a woman has straight or curly hair. A woman will have straight hair if the cortex is cylindrical or round and curly hair if it is oval.

913

Q Why do some women experience thinning hair after having a baby?

A Hormonal changes in the body can alter hair growth. A hormonal change can cause more hairs than usual to go into a rest phase that can last for months or longer. The follicles are not gone; they are just not dividing. Some women see similar hair changes when they start or stop taking birth control pills or begin the menopause process.

914

Q What is dandruff?

A Dandruff occurs when skin cells flake off the scalp. The flaking is natural and happens all over the body. On the scalp, however, larger flakes can mix with oil and dust to form dandruff. Dandruff cannot be cured but can be controlled. There are a number of shampoos that help with daily control. There is an indication that some forms of dandruff are due to a special type of yeast infection of the hair follicles. There are antiyeast shampoos available by prescription.

915

Q How do you choose a dandruff shampoo?

A The best dandruff shampoo is one that contains zinc pyrithione. In addition, salicylic acid and coal tar products are good. If over-the-counter medicated shampoos don't help, an evaluation by a dermatologist may be warranted.

916

Q Is it dangerous to get a permanent?

A Even though permanents are generally safe, overexposure can cause irritation of the scalp and dry the hair.

917

Q Do hair conditioners really work?

A Hair conditioners coat the outside of the hair shaft to make it smoother. Because hair is composed of dead cells, nothing can make a permanent change.

918

Q What does permanent hair color mean?

A Permanent hair color chemicals open the outer layer of the hair cells, the cuticle, to allow bleaching agents to take out the natural color. A new color can then be applied. If not used correctly, these types of products can damage the hair.

919

Q What are temporary hair dyes?

A Temporary dyes paint over the natural color of the hair but don't penetrate the shaft of the hair. The color gradually fades with each hair washing because it did not penetrate into the hair shaft.

920

Q Can hair dyes cause cancer?

A Some studies have shown an increased risk of non-Hodgkin's lymphoma, leukemia, and ovarian cancer from the use of hair dye. More studies will be necessary to clarify the risks of using hair dye. In the interim, it's important that hair stylists use gloves and apply the products in a well-ventilated room.

921

Q What would cause a woman to get a bald spot on the top of her head?

A Sometimes hair loss in a specific spot is due to a repeated style of wearing the hair that might cause pulling, which will break hair near the scalp. Localized hair loss, alopecia areata, has no known cause but may be immunological. However, hair will return in about 90 percent of the cases. Dermatologists will sometimes inject the area with steroids to alleviate any inflammation.

922

Q Is there any significance to pale nail beds?

A The pink tinge is a result of blood vessels in the nail bed. People who are anemic have pale nail beds. A doctor should be seen for an evaluation if a woman experiences fatigue or dizziness as well.

923

Q What causes the edge of the fingernail to become swollen and red?

A Bacterial infections of the fingernail or toenail are not uncommon and are called a paronychia. Antibiotics may stop the infection if caught early. However, an abscess or collection of pus may occur in the nail bed and should be drained and treated with antibiotics. A health-care provider should be seen for this type of condition.

924

Q What causes ingrown toenails?

A The edges of the toenail usually grow faster than the middle. Therefore, the edges tend to turn in and grow into the tender nail bed. This problem is made worse when a woman wears poorly fitted shoes with a narrow toe and high heels. A low-heeled, wide-toed shoe is helpful in prevention.

925

Q How are ingrown toe nails treated?

A Cutting the nail straight across and putting tiny pieces of sterile cotton under the edges may help if an infection has not occurred. The cotton should be changed daily. A doctor or podiatrist should be contacted if there are signs of infection.

926

Q What will make nails grow faster?

A Nails, like hair, are composed of dead cells that grow from an area of living cells beneath the cuticle. Coating the nails with polish or "nail growth" products may help avoid trauma or damage to the nail. However, since none of the products reach the nail growth matrix, they can't alter nail growth. Nails grow faster in warm weather and may be stimulated by filing or clipping. In addition, nails of people in good health grow faster than the nails of people who are ill.

927

Q Should a woman trim or push back her cuticles?

A The cuticle protects the living cell matrix that makes the nail. Trimming the cuticle or pushing it back too much can encourage an infection with bacteria or fungi. Cuticle scissors or a stick to push back the cuticle should be avoided. The best way to control cuticles is to simply remove the dead skin from the nails after a shower with a bath towel or washcloth.

928

Q What's the best way to protect nails?

A Household detergents and prolonged use in water are harmful to nails. Waterproof gloves, that are kept dry inside to prevent fungus from growing, will protect the nails from water and household chemical products. Cotton gloves can be worn at other times to protect the nail and nail bed from harm.

929

Q Are regular manicures and pedicures necessary?

A Although good nail care decreases hangnails, manicures or pedicures do not promote nail growth. If you do choose to have a manicure or pedicure, it is important to select a technician that sterilizes instruments with heat to prevent infection.

930

Q What type of nail polish is the best?

A Some women develop an allergy to the formaldehyde in certain nail products. If a rash develops around the nail or the nail starts to separate, stop using the product. Stop the polish above the cuticle to avoid polish going over the living tissue of the nail. Use nail polish remover as little as possible because overuse can damage the nail.

931

Q Are artificial nails safe?

A There can be several risks to using artificial tips or nails. One risk is an allergy to the glues, which contain a form of formaldehyde and other chemicals. In some cases, the area underneath the tips and gaps at the nail bed can trap moisture and promote fungal infections. Some women have lost nails from the infections. See a dermatologist immediately if there are signs of allergy or infection.

932

Q How fast do fingernails grow?

A The average fingernail grows about one-eighth of an inch per month. It takes about six months to replace an entire nail.

933

Q What are the white spots that occur underneath my fingernails?

A The cause of these spots is unknown, but they usually disappear with time and don't seem to damage the nail or nail bed.

934

Q What causes dry, brittle, and splitting nails?

A Damage from chores such as dishwashing or gardening can cause these types of nail problems. Nail-hardening products that are promoted to help the problem often make it worse. If the symptoms are severe, a doctor can determine if it is a result of a low thyroid function.

935

Q How is a nail fungus treated?

A Local treatment of the nail with solutions or soaks is rarely effective in treating nail fungal infections. Oral antifungal drugs are the most effective treatment. Sporonox, a relatively new medication, is effective but must be monitored by a physician. Side effects can include liver abnormalities, rash, headache, and confusion. Treatment must continue for quite some time to allow resolution of the infection and prevent recurrence.

Teeth

936

Q What can cause teeth to be stained and discolored?

A Teeth can become stained from certain foods, tobacco, red wine, and excess fluoride in the water. If a pregnant woman takes tetracycline, an antibiotic, her unborn baby's teeth may develop discolored.

937

Q How can a woman make her teeth whiter?

A The over-the-counter teeth bleaching products are not very effective. These products use a bleaching agent that is placed in a mouth plate that fits over the teeth. The mouth plate isn't custom-made, and the bleaching agent may leak. The bleaching agent is a hydrogen peroxide formulation that can help superficially stained teeth. A dentist uses a custom-made mouth plate and stronger solution that is not available as an over-the-counter product. Teeth bleaches appear to be safe although they sometimes cause temporary gum irritation. Opalescence, a patented sustained-release whitening gel available only from a dentist, is an excellent whitening agent. Laser whitening is also effective but is considerably more expensive.

938

Q How important is it to see a dentist regularly?

A Everyone should see a dentist regularly. Anyone, at any age, can get cavities. In addition to checking for gum disease and tooth problems, a dentist can detect mouth and tongue cancers. Dentists can also see problems in a woman's teeth that result from ongoing bulimic behavior.

939

Q What is a root canal?

A If the root of a tooth is damaged or infected, the underlining bone will also be affected. In a root canal, the dentist removes the nerve from the affected tooth and fills the core of the tooth. A cap is then placed over the entire remains of the tooth to protect it from breakage.

940

Q Why are crowns sometimes put on teeth?

A Teeth that are cracked, severely decayed, or already have a variety of fillings may not be able to hold another. A crown is also necessary after a root canal. The dentist will make an impression of the current tooth to make a crown that will exactly fit the tooth and surrounding area. A temporary cover will be placed on the tooth until the permanent crown is made at a laboratory. New computer programs have been developed, but are not yet widely available, to produce a permanent crown at the first visit, making a temporary crown unnecessary.

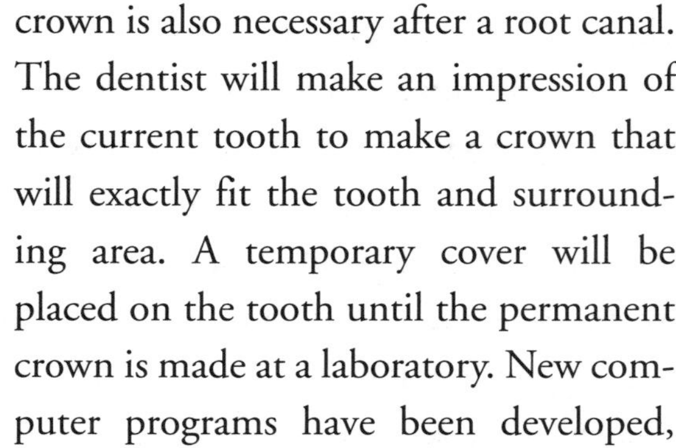

941

Q What is bonding used for?

A Bonds are acrylic resins that are used to repair broken teeth. These tooth-colored preparations are applied to damaged areas. The bonding is subject to wear and tear and must be replaced over time.

942

Q What are tooth veneers?

A Tooth veneers are to teeth as false fingernails are to fingers. These thin tooth caps can permanently cover stained or discolored teeth that don't respond to routine bleaching. They can also fill in excess space or gaps between front teeth. Veneers are custom made to fit each woman's teeth perfectly.

943

Q How can a woman avoid losing her teeth?

A There are several issues that play a part in a woman keeping her natural teeth. Good dental hygiene, brushing at least twice a day, and using dental floss are important supplements to dental visits twice a year for professional cleaning. Good nutrition cannot be overlooked to build a healthy bone structure and keep gums strong.

944

Q What is gum disease?

A Periodontal disease is the main cause of tooth loss for those over thirty-five years old. It is more likely in smokers and may run in families. Poor dental hygiene accelerates the severity of the disease. The first stage of the disease is gingivitis and is an inflammation of the gums caused by bacteria. The last stage is periodontitis, where the gums separate from the teeth and pockets of bacteria and pus form in the area.

945

Q How does gum disease cause tooth loss?

A The inflammation from the gum disease erodes the ligaments that hold the teeth in place. The teeth get loose and eventually fall out.

946

Q What are the symptoms of gum disease?

A Gum disease causes tender, swollen gums that bleed easily. There is increased sensitivity of the teeth due to recession of the gums. The person often complains of bad breath and a bad taste in the mouth.

947

Q How is gum disease treated?

A Frequent cleaning by a dental hygienist every three months and meticulous home dental care are the most important factors in controlling gum disease. Gum surgery may be necessary to remove pockets of bacteria and pus. Sometimes gum grafting can help to repair gum that has been lost.

948

Q If a woman loses one back tooth, does it need to be replaced?

A A woman's teeth will shift if the space from a lost tooth is not filled. A bridge or implant replacement will alleviate any problems that might occur from the shifting teeth such as a misalignment of the jaw, difficulty chewing, or large spaces between the teeth.

949

Q How often do dentures need to be replaced?

A Dentures will last from six months to five years depending on the care they are given and how they are made. If the woman's jaw structure changes, new dentures will have to be made regardless of their condition.

950

Q Does everyone with dentures have to use a dental adhesive?

A Adhesives are used if the dentures don't fit correctly. It is healthier to replace a poor set of dentures than use the over-the-counter adhesives.

951

Q What can be done if a woman can't get a pair of dentures to fit well?

A If a person has lost too much bone in her jaw, she will be unable to hold a denture properly in her mouth. The best treatment, in this case, is to have metallic supports placed into the jaw to hold the dentures. This procedure should be performed by an oral surgeon.

952

Q What is a dental bridge?

A A bridge is made of a maximum of four front teeth or two back teeth. It is used in the mouth to fill in the gaps left by lost teeth. A fixed metal support is anchored to healthy teeth using a cap that is attached to the bridge at each end. The healthy end support teeth are prepared for a cap that is cemented on the end teeth and attached to the bridge.

953

Q What are dental implants?

A Dental implants are false teeth that are separately fixed or anchored into the bone of the jaw. The woman having implants has to have healthy gums and bones. Metal shafts are placed into the jawbone and allowed to heal for several months. The teeth are then anchored to metal pins that fit into the sockets attached to the bone. It is important to maintain excellent dental hygiene around the implants to prevent gum disease or infection. This is a long and expensive process that takes a number of months to complete.

954

Q What are the benefits to having implants?

A Dental implants are more natural in appearance than dentures. They stay in the mouth permanently and don't have to be removed for cleaning or to sleep. The implants more closely mimic real teeth and help to preserve the strength of the jawbone. Implants can be used in children who have lost a tooth due to injury.

955

Q What are the risks of dental implants?

A There are multiple oral surgery procedures necessary for permanent dental implants. There are risks of infection at the operative site or, more seriously, into the jawbone (osteomyelitis). A bone infection may take months to treat and may not be cured until the metal anchoring plate is removed from the bone.

956

Q How does a woman choose a good dentist?

A Call the county dental society for the names of licensed dentists in your neighborhood. Often friends and neighbors are good sources of information. A family physician can also recommend a dentist. Some dental insurance companies will dictate specific dentists that have to be used.

957

Q What should a woman do if she can't afford to go to the dentist?

A Check with a local dental school to see if they are willing to do an evaluation of your dental problems. Dental students will perform the work while they are supervised by an experienced dental staff member.

958

Q What type of toothbrush should a woman use?

A A soft toothbrush that will clean the teeth and stimulate the gums without damage or irritation is the best one to use. Some people find that certain toothbrush shapes fit their mouths better than others. This is a personal decision. The most important thing about a brush, however, is that it gets used at least twice a day.

959

Q What's the difference between an oral surgeon and a dentist?

A Oral surgeons complete a two-year training program in dental surgery after dental school. They are qualified to perform surgery on the jaw, teeth, and gums and have surgical privileges at a hospital. A general dentist does not perform this type of surgery.

960

Q What type of toothpaste is the best?

A There is no evidence that one type of fluoride toothpaste is better than another. It is important, however, that it does not contain an abrasive, which can damage tooth enamel, and that it tastes good enough to use frequently.

961

Q What can a woman do if her teeth are sensitive to cold?

A Sometimes sensitivity to cold is a sign of significant dental disease. Brushing with Sensodyne toothpaste can significantly decrease the sensitivity of teeth. If the symptom persists, an evaluation by a dentist is necessary.

962

Q What is an orthodontist?

A An orthodontist is a dentist who specializes in straightening teeth and correcting abnormal jaw alignments using braces.

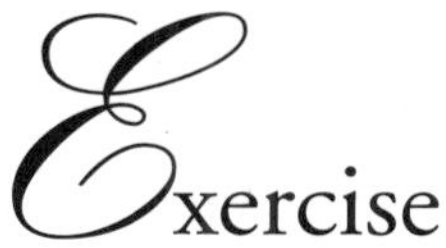

Exercise

963

Q Should a woman see a doctor before starting an exercise program?

A If a woman has been sedentary and is over the age of forty-five, it's wise to seek a checkup before starting a regular exercise program. If there are additional risk factors, such as high blood pressure, diabetes, heart disease, connective tissue disorder, or fibromyalgia, a health-care provider should monitor the program and the body's reaction.

964

Q How much exercise does a woman really need?

A To achieve cardiac fitness, a moderate aerobic exercise such as fitness walking should be done thirty to forty minutes, three to four days a week. If a woman is overweight and wants to decrease body fat, exercising daily is preferred not only to burn calories but also to temporarily increase metabolism. People who suffer from depression or anxiety disorder will benefit from daily exercise to improve overall mood.

965

Q Does a woman need to lift weights or use some type of exercise machine?

A Aerobic exercise improves the condition of the heart, increases energy, and helps to decrease body fat but doesn't increase muscle strength much. Weight lifting increases muscle mass and strength. The more muscle mass, the greater the metabolism. Both types of exercise work well together.

966

Q What is the best exercise for a woman in her forties?

A If a woman is just starting to exercise, walking is inexpensive, low risk, and very effective. Other good activities include biking or using steppers or cross-country ski machines. The risk of knee injury is high with running. Water aerobics provides an excellent cardiovascular workout. When choosing an exercise class, select one designed for women over forty just starting out. Many women who start aggressive classes and aren't in good condition risk hurting themselves.

967

Q Is it too late for a seventy-year-old woman to start an exercise program?

A Start slowly with a walking or water aerobics program. Be consistent but don't push too hard. Gradually increase the length of exercise time before increasing the intensity. It's never too late to start.

968

Q What is a good way to find an exercise class that doesn't cost a fortune?

A There are many community groups that offer low-cost exercise classes. Check the local senior citizen centers, community recreation programs, local colleges, YMCA, and churches or synagogues. A self-motivated woman will come up with a regimen that can be accomplished by walking at the local mall or college track.

969

Q What credentials should a woman look for from a personal instructor or trainer?

A A trainer will design a workout program, motivate the woman, and monitor progress. A health or athletic club can usually recommend someone they have confidence in. Ask for certifications and references from anyone who is advising you on a fitness program.

970

Q How heavy should the weights be, and how often should they be used for the best results?

A Choosing the best type of weight-lifting program depends on the age of the woman, her general health, and the desired results. A weight should be chosen that can be moved with modest effort. The exercise should be repeated enough times to make the muscle feel tired. It is important to start slowly to avoid muscle, ligament, and tendon problems. The heavier the weight, the greater the risk of injury. It's not good to exercise a muscle group more often than every forty-eight hours.

The muscle needs time to recover. Generally light weights and multiple repetitions give good results with less risk.

971

Q How can a woman tell if she's overtraining?

A People who are in good physical condition feel good and have increased energy. People who overtrain are stressing the body and don't feel well. Too much stress, training, or physical activity causes the body to break down and become ill.

972

Q How can a woman tell if she's straining a muscle?

A Muscles that are being overused or damaged by activity hurt. There is a difference between being sore after a workout and experiencing pain. An injury will hurt longer than a day or two and may feel more like a sharp burning pain. Slight soreness that quickly resolves is not worrisome. Pain that isn't relieved after a few days of rest and ibuprofen or naproxen sodium should be checked by a health-care provider.

973

Q How much water should a woman drink when she is exercising?

A The body requires six to eight glasses of water on a normal day. More is required with exercise. Even though the body doesn't always crave fluid until it is close to being dehydrated, it's crucial to good health to replace body fluids that are lost from physical activity.

974

Q Are there any moderate exercise programs a woman can continue regardless of her age?

A Walking is always a good exercise that can be modified in intensity to meet a woman's needs at any age. Another option is tai chi, which is an Asian exercise that is done in a very slow, smooth rhythm. It was originally designed as a form of meditation. Studies in older people have shown that it improves balance and muscle strength. People who practice tai chi are less likely to fall and break a bone as they get older. This type of exercise requires instruction. Lessons are available in most metropolitan areas.

975

Q Won't a woman start to look masculine if she lifts weights to increase muscle strength?

A A woman has to work out with large weights many hours a day to develop muscles similar to those men have. A woman will, however, develop firm muscle definition. Woman who have unusually large muscles may be taking high doses of male hormones.

976

Q Is it necessary to wear a special type of bra while you exercise?

A Women should wear a sports bra that provides support during exercise. Bouncing or jumping should not affect the breasts if a bra is designed for those types of activities.

977

Q What causes a woman to get tired and short of breath when she exercises?

A A woman should experience mild shortness of breath and mild fatigue after exercising. If there is continued fatigue after a brief rest period, the exercise intensity may be too hard. Shortness of breath may be a result of being out of shape, exercise-induced asthma, or a heart problem. A doctor should be consulted about these symptoms before any exercise program is continued.

978

Q How can a woman make exercising more entertaining?

A Working out with a buddy is always better than going it alone. Even if you are walking in the neighborhood, this could be your special time or time with a friend. Take along headphones and a tape if you walk alone. You can listen to music or even a book on tape.

979

Q What is cross training?

A Many women like to be active five to six days a week for energy and weight control. The concept of cross training is to rotate several different activities that use different muscle sets. A woman might alternate fitness walking, biking, and working with weights to provide the best fitness level with the least chance of injury.

980

Q Should a pregnant woman exercise?

A A healthy woman should exercise during her entire pregnancy as long as she doesn't experience any complications. Fitness walking is an excellent choice of exercise during pregnancy, as are swimming and water aerobics. It may be necessary to modify the exercise program the last three months of pregnancy to allow the blood flow needs of the placenta to take priority. Always discuss an exercise program with a health-care provider.

981

Q Should a woman do certain types of exercises when she's pregnant?

A Certain types of exercises help strengthen the pelvic floor and can be learned in a childbirth exercise class. The American College of Obstetrics and Gynecology recommends that pregnant women not do full sit-ups, double leg raises, and deep knee bends. They also suggest avoiding jerky or high-impact activities. Lying on the back for an extended period of time after the fifth month of pregnancy may decrease blood flow to the uterus.

982

Q How much exercise is necessary for good health?

A It is best to be consistent rather than intensive with an exercise program. A two- to three-mile walk, aerobics, or bike ride four times a week will keep the body in a healthy condition.

983

Q How can a woman determine her target heart rate to monitor the intensity of her exercise?

A Some exercise experts recommend monitoring the heart rate during exercise to see if the intensity of the exercise is too high or too low. To determine a maximum heart rate, a woman should subtract her age from 220. For example, a fifty-year-old woman should have a maximum heart rate of 170 beats per minute. For the maximum effect from exercise, a woman should increase her heart rate to about 75 percent of one hundred seventy, which is about 128 beats per minute. This concept of target heart rate won't work for all women. Some people naturally have a slower heart rate than others.

984

Q Is there another way to monitor the heart rate without subtracting and multiplying numbers?

A Researchers monitored women who were exercising and found that if a woman thought she had a good workout, was sweating, and mildly tired but not exhausted, that she had indeed completed adequate exercise. In other words, perception of how much a woman has exercised is probably an accurate assessment.

Quality of Life

985

Q What is body image?

A Body image is the inner perception of our outer selves. It is how a woman thinks she looks. Women with eating disorders have a distorted body image. Anorexic women, for example, may be completely emaciated but see themselves as fat.

986

Q How can a woman find time for herself when she doesn't have a minute to spare between work and family?

A Women often have trouble finding time to care for their own needs. It is crucial to make time. As women we need to learn to delegate not only at work but also in the home. Children learn by doing. We actually rob them of experiences when we jump in to help on a regular basis. Just five or ten minutes a day to be alone will help the body and mind to focus.

987

Q How does a woman manage caring for an elderly parent while also caring for her family and working full time?

A Before it becomes a monumental task that affects our own well being and that of our family, we must begin to ask for help. Many women are tormented by the thought of moving a parent to a retirement facility. However, it is important to avoid isolation and depression as people get older. A good facility will include day and evening activities to help them cope with their new life and alleviate the ongoing emotional, aging issues. Perhaps a day program for the elderly would be a compromise. Role reversal is a difficult task. Look for help from support groups in your community.

988

Q What can a woman do to help herself and her children feel more comfortable about the idea of their being alone at home after school?

A If your children have a set time to call you at work after school, you will gain peace of mind and they will learn commitment. This is an excellent time for children to learn responsibility through specific chores that need to be done each day. Post emergency phone numbers and make arrangements with an adult in the neighborhood to step in at a moment's notice in case of an emergency.

989

Q How can a woman get more energy when she's always tired?

A It sounds strange to say exercise or body movement when the mind and thoughts say you're too tired. However, exercise is a natural antidepressant. The smallest amount of movement you can accomplish will help the body to be energized. Be realistic about what you have scheduled and look objectively to see if anyone could possibly accomplish it in one day. If none of these ideas work, have a medical evaluation. Something else could be causing your fatigue.

990

Q Is there anything available for those of us who can't afford a makeover or day spa?

A Take a day off from work or home activities and treat yourself to a lunch out. Take advantage of the stores that have makeup artists or special product showings where they will do a facial or makeover at no cost. You are under no obligation to buy anything and have enjoyed a day of pampering. With a little creativity, you can have a great day at minimal cost.

991

Q What can a woman do to stop smoking when she's been doing it since she was a teenager?

A Your health-care provider can give you a prescription for a patch or you might use the nicotine gum to help with physical withdrawal symptoms. Being with other people in a group situation may be the answer to some of the psychological problems that arise from not practicing an addiction. Look in the phone book for a group like Smoke Enders or Nicotine Anonymous. Some women find hypnosis or acupuncture to be helpful.

992

Q How can a woman talk to her partner comfortably about prior sexual contacts?

A Few situations are as intimate as having sex with someone. Start by saying how difficult it is to talk about sex but assure your partner that you want the relationship to be safe and fulfilling. Share your own sexual history including diseases, if any, and let your partner know that you want to be very careful about protecting your health. Ask about IV drug use and any sexually transmitted diseases before any intercourse is agreed to. It's a major decision to choose a sexual partner. Take some extra time before turning a friendship into a sexual relationship.

993

Q What can a woman do to feel more comfortable when asking her doctor embarrassing health questions?

A Keep in mind that your health-care provider is trained to talk about the sexual concerns and problems most women experience. Begin by talking about how hard it is and how embarrassed you are, and the nervousness will quickly disappear. The health-care provider should encourage questions and put you at ease.

994

Q What can a woman do at home to survive a cold?

A Treating cold symptoms with a pain reliever and decongestant will help. Increased rest will help the body produce more interferon, which is a natural antiviral drug. Medical research confirms that chicken soup helps decrease the length and severity of an upper respiratory viral infection. Vitamin C may help decrease the length or severity of viral infections.

995

Q With everyone keeping such tight schedules, is sleep deprivation at a new high?

A Sleep disorders are related to aging and depression. And as our population ages, so will some of the related disorders. Early awakening is a common sign of depression. There are sleep laboratories at many hospitals across the country that can make an evaluation by monitoring you while you sleep. It's well documented that people with a regular exercise program sleep better than those who are sedentary. Some helpful hints to get a good night's sleep include a regular bedtime routine, quiet time or a period of meditation, and a warm bath. Sleeping pills can be addictive. The safest prescription pill is Restoril. Benedryl is an over-the-counter antihistamine but can be used as a sleep aid periodically. Several herbal formulations found in a health food store are recommended to aid sleep. It's important not to stay in bed when you wake up in the middle of the night. Get up and do something boring.

996

Q What's the difference between an underarm deodorant and antiperspirant?

A Sweat has no smell. Odor develops when bacteria start to interact with sweat. Therefore, a product that decreases the bacteria will decrease odor. An antiperspirant uses aluminum compounds to decrease the amount of perspiration. A deodorant focuses on odor elimination rather than perspiration.

997

Q How common is incest?

A Incest is more common in our society than people think. One in four women report some type of forced sexual activity prior to the age of eighteen, and at least 10 percent of this abuse is incestuous. Women who are abused as children have a much higher incidence of depression, eating disorders, and substance abuse.

998

Q Is domestic violence becoming more common?

A The incidence of domestic abuse or violence, physical and psychological, is extremely high. One in seven women who visit a physician and one in three women seen in an emergency room have suffered abuse at the hands of a spouse. Women who see their physicians often for many non-specific complaints have a much higher rate of abuse than women who go yearly for a routine physical. Women who have stories to cover a bruise or broken bone repeatedly indicate to health providers they are in trouble. Women tend to stay in a violent situation because they don't feel deserving or worthy enough to be treated well. The abuser will follow each episode of battering with apologies, making the woman believe it will never happen again. A local hospital can provide any woman with the name and phone number of an area battered women's shelter.

999

Q What motivates one person to rape another?

A Rape is about violence, not about sex. The rapist wants to dominate or humiliate the other person. Rape is the weapon rather than a knife or gun. At least 10 percent of women in the United States have been raped and up to 50 percent have been threatened with it. If a woman is raped, she should seek immediate medical attention even if she doesn't feel injured. Most major hospital emergency rooms will have a team on call to meet the needs of rape victims. A woman should not shower, bathe, or douche before going to the emergency room. She should take an extra change of clothes in case the clothes she was wearing are kept as evidence. The local rape crisis center will be helpful for support group and counselor referrals.

To protect against rape, it's important to pay attention to surroundings when walking outside the home whether it's daytime or evening. Park in well-lit areas at night, keep keys in your hand, and pay attention. A self-defense course might instill confidence in a woman. Keep doors and windows at home locked and be careful about inviting people you don't know well into your home. If you feel uncomfortable in a situation, trust your instincts and get out. Most rape situations involve someone you know.

1000

Q Why do some people wear metal allergy bracelets?

A People with allergies that result in serious reaction, or with diseases such as epilepsy, asthma, or diabetes, should strongly consider wearing a medical alert bracelet or necklace. In case of an accident, the medical provider will have this vital information if the person cannot talk. It's also important to carry a wallet card with the same information.

Resources

American Anorexic/Bulimia Association
Suite 1R
293 Central Park West
New York, NY 10024
212-501-8351

American Council for Drug Education
136 East 64 Street
New York, NY 10021
800-488-3784

American Diabetes Association, Inc.
1660 Duke Street
Alexandria, VA 22314-3427
800-232-3472

American Lung Association
1740 Broadway
New York, NY 10019-4374
212-315-8700

American Psychiatric Association
Code HUP
Division of Public Affairs
1400 K Street, NW
Washington, DC 20005
202-682-6000

Arthritis Foundation
1314 Spring Street NW
Atlanta, GA 30309
404-872-7100
March of Dimes Foundation
White Plains, NY 10605
800-367-6630

National Cancer Institute
Build 31
Bethesda, MD 20892
800-422-6237

National Coalition Against Domestic Violence
PO Box 18749
Denver, CO 80218
303-839-1852

National Institute on Aging
PO Box 8057
Gaithersburg, MD 20898-8057
800-222-2225

National Institute of Mental Health
5600 Fishers Lane
Rockville, MD 20857
800-421-4211

National Osteoporosis Foundation
Suite 500
1150 17th Street, NW
Washington, DC 20036-4603
202-223-2226

National Women's Health Network
514 10th Street, NW
Washington, DC 20004
202-347-1140

Office of Alternative Medicine
National Institutes of Health
Suite 450
6120 Executive Boulevard
Rockville, MD 20892-9904
301-402-2466

Planned Parenthood Federation of America
810 Seventh Avenue
New York, NY 10019
800-829-7732 (abortion information)
800-230-7526 (clinic referrals)

Susan G. Komen Breast Cancer Foundation
Suite 370
5005 LBJ Freeway
Dallas, TX 75244
800-I'M AWARE
800-462-9273

Abortion and Reproductive Rights Internet Resources
http://www.caral.org/abortion.html

Action on Smoking and Health (ASH) (national legal-action antismoking organization)
http://ash.org/

American Academy of Family Physicians
http://www.aafp.org/

American Board of Obstetrics and Gynecology
http://www.metronet.com/~rhino/

American Cancer Society
http://www.cancer.org/smokeout/

American College of Obstetricians and Gynecologists
http://www.acog.com

American Heart Association
http://www.amhrt.org/

American Lung Association
http://www.lungusa.org/

American Medical Association
http://www.ama-assn.org/

American Medical Women's Association
http://www.amwa-doc.org/

American Society for Reproductive Medicine
http://www.asrm.com/

Avicenna Medline Access
http://www.avicenna.com/

Bandolier
http://www.jr2.ox.ac.uk/Bandolier/

Centers for Disease Control & Prevention, National Center for Chronic Disease Prevention and Health Promotion, Office of Smoking and Health
http://www.cdc.gov/nccdphp/osh/tobacco.htm

Centre for Evidence-Based Medicine
http://cebm.jr2.ox.ac.uk/docs/adminpage.html

Cochrane Collaboration
http://hiru.mcmaster.ca/cochrane/default.htm

DOC (Doctors Ought to Care)
http://www.bcm.tmc.edu/doc/

Dr. Felix's Free MEDLINE Page, in collaboration with Docnet
http://195.152.9.7:80/drfelix

Evidence-Based Medicine
http://www.acponline.org/journals/catnew/journal/journals1.htm

Food and Drug Administration Home Page
http://www.fda.gov/

Hardin Meta Directory-Obstetrics, Gynecology and Women's Health
http://www.arcade.uiowa.edu/hardin_www/md-obgyn.html

Housecall Medline Access
http://pressconf.housecall.com/prologin.html

healthfinder-a gateway consumer health information website from the U.S. government
http://www.healthfinder.gov

HealthGate Medline
http://www.healthgate.com/HealthGate/MEDLINE/search.shtml

Healthtouch-Online for better health
http://www.healthtouch.com/level1/menu.htm

Healthworks Medline Access
http://www.healthworks.co.uk/hw/medline/registermed.html

Healthy.Net-MEDLINE Search
http://www.healthworld.com/library/search/medline.htm

Helix Medline Access
http://www/HELIX.com/

In Your Corner, Health and Wellness Products
www.inyourcorner.com

Infotrieve Medline Service Provider
http://www.infotrieve.com/

Internet Grateful Med Medline Search
http://igm.nlm.nih.gov/

Johathon Tward's Multimedia Medical Reference Library Search and Medline
http://www.tiac.net/users/jtward/search.htm#medline

Knight-Ridder Information Web Site
http://www.dialog.com/#start

Knowledge Finder
http://www.kfinder.com/medline_test.html

Library of Congress Home Page
http://ftp.loc.gov/

McMaster University EBM Informatics
http://hiru.mcmaster.ca/ebm/

Medline Database at Community of Science, Inc.
http://muscat.gdb.org/repos/medl

Medline URLs for Medical Matrix Sites
http://www.medmatrix.org/info/medlinetable.html)

Medscape Medline Search
http://www.medscape.com/textSearch.form.fcgi

MedWeb: Gynecology and women's health
http://www.gen.emory.edu/medweb/medweb.gynecology.html

MD Answers at SilverPlatter
http://php2.silverplatter.com/physicians/

NCEMCH Home Page
http://www.ncemch.georgetown.edu/

NetWellness Home Page
http://ovchin.uc.edu/

OBGYN.net
http://www.obgyn.net

NlightN Medline Search
http://www.nlightn.com/

NLM's PubMed Medline Retrieval System
http://www4.ncbi.nim.nih.gov/PubMed/

OBGYN.net-The Obstetrics and Gynecology Network
http://www.obgyn.net/home.htm

OncoLink, The University of Pennsylvania Cancer Center Resouce
http://cancer.med.upenn.edu/

Ovid On Call Medline and Medical Databases
http://preview.ovid.com/libpreview/

Paper Chase Medical Literature Searching
http://enterprise.bih.harvard.edu/paper-chase/

PDRnetCom
http://www.pdrnet.com/

PhyNet Medline Access
http://medline.phynet.net/plwebcgi/fastweb.exe?viewform

PHYSICIANS/ ONLINE Home Page
http://www.po.com

Plymouth Area Communities Medical Access Network
http://www.pacman.org/

"Practice Guidelines, Statements and Opinions" SOGC
http://sogc.medical.org/sogc_docs/public/Guidelines.html

Prototype MEDLINE evaluation criteria (UVA):
http://www.med.virginia.edu/~wmd4n/medline.html

SCHARR-Evidence Based Medicine
http://panizzi.shef.ac.uk/auracle//links.html

The Master Anti-Smoking Page (run by Elliot Essman, a consumer)
http://www.autonomy.com/smoke.htm

The Society of Gynecologic Oncologists
http://www.sgo.org/

United Nations and other international organizations
http://www.undcp.org/unlinks.html

United States Public Health Service
http://phs.os.dhhs.gov/phs/phs.html

Washington Section of DOC
http://kickbutt.org/

WebMedline
http://www-med.standford.edu/cgi-bin/med-lookup

World Health Organization WWW Home Page
http://www.who.ch/

Index

Note: Numbers are question numbers, not page numbers.
(Boldface number indicates that the indexed topic is the primary subject of that question)

A

B

D

F

I

J

K

L

M

N

O

Q

R

T[illegible]

U

V

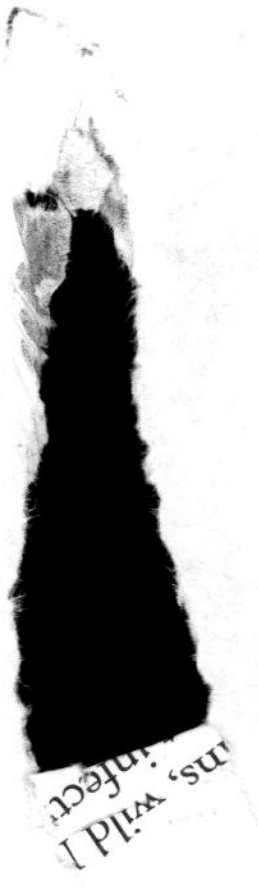